INFECTIOUS DISEASES

MEDICAL SCHOOL CRASH COURSE

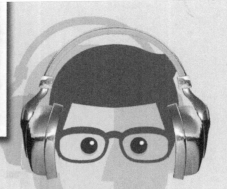

HIGH-YIELD CONTENT REVIEW

Q&A AND "KEY TAKEAWAYS"

TOP 100 TEST QUESTIONS

FOLLOW-ALONG PDF MANUAL

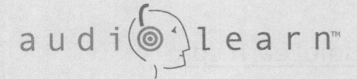

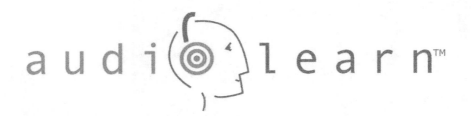

IFECTIOUS DISEASES

Medical School Crash Course™

www.AudioLearn.com

Table of Contents

Preface i

Chapter 1: The Human Immune System 1

Innate Immune System 1

Adaptive Immune System 5

Immunosuppression 8

Key Takeaways 9

Quiz 9

Chapter 2: Common Bacterial Infections 12

Cellulitis 12

Bacterial Pneumonia 12

Bacterial Gastroenteritis 14

Peritonitis 14

Sinusitis 15

Acute Otitis Media 16

Tuberculosis 18

Osteomyelitis 19

Key Takeaways 20

Quiz 20

Chapter 3: Common Viral Infections 23

Influenza 23

Upper Respiratory Infection 24

Respiratory Syncytial Virus 24

Viral Gastroenteritis 25

Viral Hepatitis 26

Epstein-Barr Viral Infections (EBV) 26

Key Takeaways 27

Quiz 27

Chapter 4: Common Fungal Infections 30

Systemic Candidiasis 30

Aspergillosis 31

Histoplasmosis 32

Cryptococcosis 34

Coccidioidomycosis 34

Blastomycosis 35

Key Takeaways 35

Quiz 36

Chapter 5: Common Protozoal Infections **38**

Malaria 38

Toxoplasmosis 40

Leishmaniasis 41

African sleeping sickness 43

Chagas disease 43

Giardiasis 45

Key Takeaways 46

Quiz 47

Chapter 6: Common Parasitic Infections **49**

Cestodiasis 49

Ascariasis 50

Filariasis 51

Scabies 53

Pediculosis Pubis 54

Pediculosis Capitus 55

Pediculosis Corporis 56

Key Takeaways 57

Quiz 57

Chapter 7: Antibiotics and Antiviral Agents **59**

Using Antibiotics in Medicine 59

Classes of Antibiotics 60

Antiviral Drugs 63

Common Antiviral Drugs 66

Amantadine 66

Relenza (zanamivir) 66

Tamiflu (oseltamivir phosphate) 66

Rapivab (peramivir) 66

Adefovir 67

Famciclovir 67

Interferon 67

Acyclovir and Valacyclovir 67

Key Takeaways 68

Quiz 68

Chapter 8: Antifungals, Anti-Protozoal Agents, and Anti-Parasitic Agents 71

Antifungal Drugs 71

Clotrimazole 71

Miconazole 72

Terbinafine 72

Fluconazole 72

Ketoconazole 73

Amphotericin B 73

Anti-Protozoal Drugs 73

Antimalarial Drugs 74

Melarsoprol 76

Eflornithine 76

Lampit (nifurtimox) 76

Suramin 76

Antihelminthic Drugs 77

Pediculosis Drugs 77

Key Takeaways 78

Quiz 78

Chapter 9: Sepsis 81

Bacterial Sepsis 81

Signs and Symptoms of Sepsis 82

Diagnosis of Sepsis 82

Treatment of Sepsis 83

Prognosis of Sepsis 84

Key Takeaways 85

Quiz 85

Chapter 10: HIV Disease 88

HIV Virus 88

HIV/AIDS 91

HIV Drugs 93

Key Takeaways 94

Quiz 94

Chapter 11: Sexually Transmitted Infections **97**

Gonorrhea 97

Chlamydia 98

Syphilis 99

Human papillomavirus 101

Herpes Simplex 102

Key Takeaways 103

Quiz 103

Chapter 12: Neglected Tropical Infections and Rare Infections **106**

Dengue Fever 106

Leprosy 107

Rabies 109

Trachoma 110

Typhus 111

Key Takeaways 112

Quiz 112

Chapter 13: Nosocomial Infections and Opportunistic Infections **115**

MRSA 115

Pneumocystis Pneumonia 116

Clostridium Difficile 117

Cytomegalovirus 118

Kaposi's Sarcoma 119

Key Takeaways 120

Quiz 120

Summary **123**

Course Questions and Answers **125**

Preface

Many different types of organisms can overwhelm the human immune system, causing various infectious diseases. Bacterial and viral diseases are extremely common, while protozoal and parasitic infections are less commonly encountered. Collectively, these disorders are primarily treated with antimicrobial medications, which are discussed in this course. Infectious diseases that merit special attention such as HIV disease, sepsis, nosocomial infections, sexually-transmitted diseases, and opportunistic infections are also covered in this course.

The human immune system represents the host defense system, which is the topic of chapter one. There are two major components to the immune system, including the innate (nonspecific) immune system and the adaptive (specific) immune system. Each of these parts of the immune system have acellular and cellular components. This chapter is intended to provide a brief outline of the innate and adaptive immune system and how they fight infectious diseases.

Common bacterial infections is the subject of chapter two in the course. There are infections that can arise spontaneously from a break in the protective barriers, such as the GI tract, respiratory tract, and skin. Viral infections may be worsened concomitant bacterial infections as the host becomes compromised by the initial viral infection. Bacteria are unicellular organisms, of which there are Gram-positive, Gram-negative, and Acid-Fast bacterial infections that can commonly occur in humans.

The subject of chapter three is common viral infections. Viral infections are more common than bacterial infections. While there are antiviral treatments for various viral infections, most viral infections spontaneously resolve due to the patient's own immune system response. Infections with viruses may be systemic or localized to a certain body area, such as the respiratory tract, liver, or gastrointestinal tract.

Chapter four coveres fungal infections. Fungal diseases range from minor to more severe diseases requiring aggressive therapy. Fungal organisms are not drastically biochemically different from human cells and more difficult to kill without significant side effects. Common fungal diseases include Aspergillosis, Candidiasis, Histoplasmosis, Cryptococcosis and Coccidiomycosis.

In chapter five there will be a comprehensive discussion of protozoal diseases. Protozoa are unicellular, eukaryotic, and non-photosynthetic organisms, of which, only a few cause human disease. Many protozoal infections are enteric in nature, leading to roughly the same symptoms from organism to organism. Other protozoal diseases, such as malaria, affect other body areas. Protozoal diseases are much more common in developing countries of the world.

In chapter six of the course, there will be a discussion of most of the human-host parasitic diseases. While protozoa are considered parasitic, this chapter will talk more on some of the other parasitic diseases, including those caused by endoparasites (which cause internal disease) and those caused by ectoparasites (which cause external human disease). Parasites are known to cause a type of human disease called a parasitosis. Most parasites don't cause any type of disease; however, there are parasites that infect just about all living organisms.

In chapter seven of the course, the topic will be antibacterial medications, known as antibiotics, and antiviral drugs. There are dozens of antibiotics that vary according to their mechanism of action against different bacterial organisms. Some antibiotics are bactericidal and kill bacteria outright, while others are bacteriostatic, meaning they only stop the growth of bacteria, requiring an intact immune system to be functional against bacterial infections. Drugs that act against viruses mainly attack an element of the life cycle of viruses, while there are a select few that act by enhancing the immune system's response against the viral organism.

Chapter eight in the course covers the broad topic of antifungal medications, anti-protozoal medications, and anti-parasitic medications. Antifungal drugs can be topical, intravenous, or oral. Anti-protozoal drugs are generally oral drugs and vary greatly depending on the protozoal organism being treated. Anti-parasitic drugs can be internally taken for things like helminthiasis or used externally for ectoparasitic diseases, such as scabies and pediculosis infestations.

Sepsis is the topic of discussion of chapter nine. It is a unique infectious disease, usually involving some type of bacteremia (which can be Gram-negative or Gram-positive sepsis) and the body's adverse reaction to the bloodborne organism. Sepsis is often accompanied by a systemic inflammatory response and multiple organ dysfunction. Many people who die of sepsis have death secondary to multiple organ failure stemming from the overwhelming inflammatory response to the infection.

The focus of chapter ten is the spectrum of HIV/AIDS and the virus behind these diseases. HIV disease is caused by the human immunodeficiency virus, which is a type of retrovirus. The disease is transferred directly from one human to another through an exchange of blood or bodily fluids. The disease is not curable; however, there are several drug regimens for HIV infections that will slow the progression of the disease.

The main topic of chapter ten is sexually transmitted infections or STIs. These are specific infectious diseases that are passed primarily from person to person through sexual activity and the exchange of bodily fluids. Many are bacterial diseases, which are curable through the use of antibiotics. Others are viral infections that cannot be cured but may be managed (in some cases) by using antiviral drugs. Several STIs are often contracted simultaneously in high risk patients, and should be tested for and treated at the same time.

Chapter twelve is about some of the more important yet neglected tropical infections and other rare infectious diseases. Mosquito-borne diseases like dengue fever are highly linked to living in or traveling to a tropical location. Other infectious processes are not necessarily seen in tropical areas but are more common in poor or rural parts of the world. Leprosy, rabies, typhus, and trachoma are rare infections that are not often seen by the practitioner in developed countries but are important to recognize and be able to treat.

The focus of chapter thirteen is opportunistic infections and nosocomial infections. These are infections that tend to be seen in patients who are hospitalized (nosocomial infections) or patients with a poor immune system (opportunistic infections). The classically immunocompromised host is one with HIV disease; however, immunocompromised patients can have other conditions or may be taking drugs that affect their immune system. Nosocomial infections can affect patients with intact immune systems who become ill because they are hospitalized and there are organisms that tend to cluster in these geographical areas.

Chapter 1: The Human Immune System

There are two major components to the human immune system, including the innate (nonspecific) immune system and the adaptive (specific) immune system. Each of these parts of the immune system have acellular (humoral) and cellular components. This chapter provides a brief outline of the innate and adaptive immune system and how they fight infectious diseases.

Innate Immune System

The innate immune system or the nonspecific immune system is an important but ancient part of the human immune system. It is evolutionarily believed to be the first immune system to be present in vertebrates and is able to fight microorganisms without specificity. There are specific cells in the human innate immune system that respond well to a pathogenic infiltration, but do not provide any long-lasting immunity to the pathogen. The innate immune system is found not only in humans but can be found in other animals and in plants. In lower order animals and plants, it is the dominant immune system found, whereas in humans, it is roughly equal in efficacy to the adaptive immune system.

There are several functions of the human innate immune system. Its first job is to release cytokines that act as chemical mediators to recruit other types of immune cells to the infection site. It then activates the complement cascade, which helps identify pathogens, activate immune cells, and promote the clearance of dead cells and antibody complexes from the area of infection. Next, the innate immune system identifies foreign substances and removes them from the body. This system is also involved in antigen presentation to the cells of the adaptive immune system. Finally, the innate immune system is acts like a physical or chemical barrier to pathogens.

The first and probably most important part of the immune system is the anatomical barrier system. The skin provides a physical barrier to pathogens and eliminates pathogens through desquamation, sweating, and the use organic acids that are toxic to pathogens. The GI tract acts to get rid of pathogens through peristalsis, secreting bile acids, gastric acid (the first line of defense), thiocyanate, digestive enzymes, and defensins. Gut flora also act to repel infectious disease. (In human breast milk, defensin play a crucial role in infant immunity.) The respiratory tract releases defensins and surfactant, and has ciliary cells that brush away pathogens. The nasopharynx has mucus, lysozyme, and saliva to repel pathogens, and the eyes produce tears to wash pathogens away.

The main barrier to pathogens is the skin and other epithelial surfaces (in the GI and respiratory tract). They form an impermeable layer of cells that pathogens just can't get into and act as the first line of defense. The act of shedding of skin and desquamation help remove bacteria and other infectious agents that have become adherent to skin cells. The lack of blood supply and the fact that the skin surface is dry helps prevent infection. Sebaceous glands secrete substances that are hostile to bacterial organisms. Both the respiratory and GI tract have mechanical ways of getting rid of pathogens using cilia and peristalsis, respectively. Mucus in both systems can trap infectious organisms. The gut flora helps by secreting toxins that kill other pathogens or by competing with other bacteria for a place in the gut flora. Tears and saliva help flush out bacteria from the mouth and eyes.

If the barriers are disrupted, inflammation is the end result and the body's first reaction to a possible infection. Inflammation is triggered by chemicals released by cells that have become injured. The act of inflammation helps establish a physical barrier against infectious diseases spreading and promotes the healing process of damaged tissue after the pathogen has been cleared out.

There are numerous cells involved in the process of acute inflammation. These include mastocytes (mast cells), Kupffer cells, histiocytes, dendritic cells, and macrophages. While they are most known for their role in allergy and anaphylaxis, mast cells play an important role in the innate immune system and closely associated with wound healing, angiogenesis, immune tolerance, defense against pathogens, and blood–brain barrier function. Kupffer cells are also known as stellate macrophages (located in the liver). Histiocytes come from bone marrow stem cells that circulate through the blood system and get into the various organs, where they differentiate into histiocytes, which are part of the mononuclear phagocytic system. Dendritic cells process antigen material and present the antigen on the cell surface to the T cells of the immune system. They are the main cellular messengers between the innate and the adaptive immune systems.

The cells of the innate immune system have pattern recognition receptors or PRRs, which can recognize the difference between pathogens and host cells by identifying pathogen-associated molecular patterns or PAMPs. When there is injury, the PRR recognizes the PAMP on the pathogen, releasing chemical inflammatory mediator that are responsible for the clinical signs of inflammation.

Inflammation is the result of certain chemical factors that are made in the inflammatory process, including prostaglandins, leukotrienes, serotonin, bradykinin, and histamine. Pain receptors are activated and there is localized vasodilatation of the arteries and veins so that blood cells can easily get to the pathogen (especially neutrophils, which travel through the bloodstream). Neutrophils are not only phagocytic, but they act to trigger other aspects of the immune system by releasing attractants that recruit more lymphocytes and leukocytes to the scene. Cytokines attract other cells and modulate the immune response.

Several important cytokines in the immune response include tumor necrosis factor (TNF), high-mobility group protein 1 (HMG-1), and interleukin-1 (IL-1). TNF is a superfamily of cytokines that can cause cell death (apoptosis). Activated macrophages and monocytes secrete HMG-1 as a type of cytokine mediator of inflammation. IL-1 plays a major role in the regulation of the immune response and in the regulation of the inflammatory response to infections or sterile injuries.

The inflammatory response leads to skin redness from an increase in blood circulation, local heat to the infected area or a systemic fever, swelling of infected tissues (as is seen in the joints in rheumatoid arthritis or skin swelling near an infection site), increased mucus production (especially in the respiratory tract), increased pain (locally or systemically), and dysfunction of the infected organs.

The complement system is an important part of the innate immune system. It involves a cascade of molecules in the immune system that complements the ability of antibodies to eliminate pathogens or marks pathogens for destruction. The complement system is mad in the liver by hepatocytes but act all over the body. The function of the complement system is to recruit new immune cells, opsonize (tag) pathogens by coating them, cause the cytolysis of pathogens (by forming holes in their plasma membrane), and helping to eliminate antigen-antibody complexes that have been neutralized.

There are three separate complement pathways that end up in basically the same way. The first is the classical pathway that starts when antibodies bind to the bacterial surface. The second is the alternative pathway that doesn't need an antibody to become active. The third is the lectin pathway, which starts whenever lectins bind to the mannose molecule on bacteria.

Figure 1 shows the activity of the complement system:

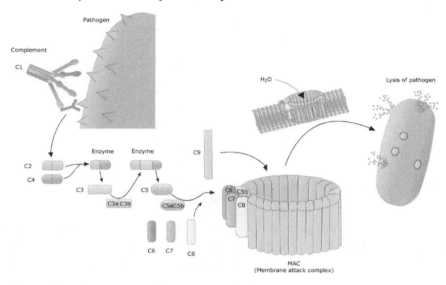

Figure 1

Leukocytes, by definition, are any kind of white blood cell. In general, leukocytes are associated with the blood and aren't necessarily associated with any particular tissue (except for the bone marrow, where they originate). They are generally free to interact with pathogens anywhere in the body (as well as foreign particles and cellular debris). Once a leukocyte is formed it has a certain half-life and doesn't divide any further (being the product of hematopoietic stem cells in the bone marrow). The basic innate-related leukocytes are natural killer cells, mast cells, eosinophils, basophils, neutrophils, macrophages, and dendritic cells. (Of these, the neutrophils, macrophages, and dendritic cells have phagocytic functions).

Mast cells are innate immune cells that live in the mucus membranes and connective tissue. As mentioned they are associated with the anaphylactic response and allergies. They are also associated with the defense against pathogens and wound healing as well. These cells are responsible for the release of hormonal mediators, heparin, and histamine as a part of the inflammatory response. They also release chemokines (chemotactic cytokines) into the inflamed area. It is histamine that is responsible for blood vessel dilatation and the typical signs of inflammation seen in an injury.

A phagocyte is any cell that "eats" an injured cell, foreign particle, or pathogenic organism. It is able to extend part of its cytoplasm outward so that it can wrap around a pathogen until it is inside the cell (inside an endosome). The endosome mixes with lysosomes, which contain enzymes and other toxic substances that destroy what has been engulfed. Phagocytes are stimulated by cytokines and are represented by dendritic cells, neutrophils, and macrophages. Phagocytes have the ability to participate in programmed cell death or apoptosis. Any dead cells are marked for destruction and are phagocytized by the phagocytic cells.

Figure 2 shows what phagocytosis schematically looks like:

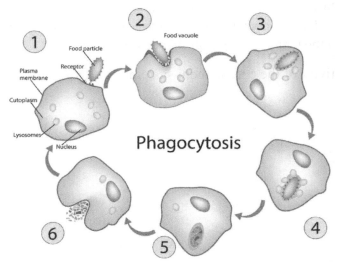

Figure 2

Macrophages are particularly large leukocytes that can move to the tissues from the bloodstream by migration across the capillary walls in order to pursue tissue-related pathogens. Monocytes are what macrophages are called when they are in the bloodstream. These represent the most effective phagocytic cells, able to phagocytize almost anything. Macrophages can release reactive oxygen species as part of a "respiratory burst", which kills pathogens nearby. They also secrete chemokines to recruit other cells to the infected site.

Neutrophils are granulocytes (along with basophils and eosinophils) because they contain visible granules in the cytoplasm. The granules inside neutrophils contain many different types of toxic substances that have the ability to kill pathogens. They are like macrophages in that the exhibit a respiratory burst (involving hydrogen peroxide, hypochlorite, and oxygen free radicals). Neutrophils represent up to 60 percent of all circulating leukocytes and are the first cells to be on site at an area of infection. About 10 billion neutrophils are made each day in the absence of infection, with up to 100 billion neutrophils made when an inflammatory process is occurring.

Dendritic cells are also phagocytic. They are located in the tissues and in close contact with the environment. Dendritic cells in the skin are known as Langerhans cells. They can also line the GI tract (stomach and intestinal walls), lung tissue, and the nose. While they look like neuronal dendrites, there is no relationship between the two. One of the main functions of dendritic cells is antigen presentation, making them a close link between the innate and adaptive immune systems.

Eosinophils and basophils are granulocytes. Basophils release histamine in response to parasites and as part of an allergic reaction. Eosinophils release toxic proteins and oxygen free radicals whenever there is a parasitic infection. They are also active during allergic reactions so their release of granules is highly regulated so they don't destroy normal tissues.

Natural killer cells or NK cells are an important component of the innate immune system. They don't attack pathogens directly but are responsible for destroying damaged or unhealthy cells, such as tumor cells or virally-infected cells. They look for a missing-self situation, when there are low levels of the MCH

I complex (major histocompatibility complex I). Low levels of MCH I are seen with viral infections. Normal cells aren't recognized by NK cells because they have lots of MCH I on their cell membranes.

Gamma/delta T cells are a subset of T cells that are on the border between the innate and the adaptive immune system. They rearrange T cell receptor genes in order to create junctional diversity and make a memory cell (this is an adaptive function). These cells also act in the innate immune system by responding directly to stressed or injured epithelial cells.

The entire innate immune response is regulated by neuronal circuits that help to control the production of cytokines. There is an inflammatory reflex that controls the cytokine activity in the spleen. There are action potentials created in the vagus nerve that mediate the release of the neurotransmitter acetylcholine, which in turn blocks the release of cytokines, decreasing inflammation.

The innate immune system responds differently to different pathogens. With viruses (which infect cells), there is mainly the activity of NK cells and phagocytosis. Most intracellular bacteria also involve NK cells and phagocytosis. Extracellular bacteria activate complement and get phagocytized. Intracellular protozoal infections are difficult because they don't activate complement and can't get phagocytized. The extracellular protozoa (like giardia and ameba infections) activate complement and get phagocytized. Extracellular fungal infections (like Candida and Histoplasma) require NK cells and complement to be destroyed.

Some pathogens have evolved in ways that allow them to evade the immune system. Mycobacterium tuberculosis replicates inside cells, which confuses the innate immune system. Salmonella creates a protective capsule that prevents lysis. Bacteroides can inhibit phagocytosis by adversely affecting the phagocytic receptors. They can also mimic host cells so they are not viewed as foreign. Staphylococcus aureus blocks the phagocyte's ability to respond to normal chemokine signals. Other bacteria (such as Bacillus anthracis, Streptococcus pyogenes, and tuberculosis) can directly kill phagocytes. Certain chronic infections (like Pseudomonas) will make biofilms that protect the organisms from innate cell invasion.

Viral infections are partly dealt with by the secretion of type 1 interferons by dendritic cells. Immune cells recognize the different types of nucleic acids seen in viruses (like double-stranded RNA). Viruses can affect this process by interfering with interferon production. Viruses can produce proteins that block interferon or can block the process necessary to make interferon.

Adaptive Immune System

The adaptive immune system is also referred to as the specific immune system or the acquired immune system. It is evolutionarily younger than the innate immune system and creates a type of immunological memory after being exposed to a specific pathogen, leading to an enhancement of the immune response whenever the pathogen enters the body at a later time. Once the adaptive immune system has done its job, the individual is always protected from the infection (except in some cases, such as the chickenpox virus). The adaptive cells can destroy toxic molecules made by the pathogens as well as the pathogens themselves. When the body can't tell the difference between harmful and harmless antigens, things like allergies occur. When the body can't tell the difference between self- and non-self-antigens, the end result is an autoimmune disease. The main cells of the adaptive immune system are the lymphocytes (divided into B cells and T cells). The B cells are responsible for producing antibodies (immunoglobulins). The antibodies inactivate the antigen, allowing for the antigen to be destroyed.

The receptors that are connected to the adaptive immune system are gradually acquired during the human lifespan (which is not the case in the innate immune system). When it is adaptive, it prepares the body's immune system for future invasions, while it can be maladaptive in autoimmune situations. Memory B cells and memory T cells contribute to long-lasting and highly specific immunity.

The adaptive immune system kicks in when the innate immune system fails or when a certain threshold level of antigen is reached. The dendritic cell can present antigens to the adaptive immune cells. The main function of the adaptive immune system is to recognize self and non-self-antigens as part of antigen presentation. It also generates cellular responses that eliminate pathogens or pathogen-containing cells and helps develop immunological memory through memory cells (T cells and B cells).

The main cells of the adaptive immune system are the T lymphocytes and the B lymphocytes. Together, these represent 20-40 percent of WBCs circulating in the system (mostly in the tissues or lymphatic system). Both T cells and B cells come from the same type of multipotent hematopoietic stem cells and look the same until they are activated. B cells play a big role in humoral immunity, while T cells play a big role in cell-mediated immunity.

The T cells are immature when released by the bone marrow and then travel to the thymus where they become immature thymocytes and differentiate into T cells. The lymphocyte pool circulates continuously in the body so that antigen-specific lymphocytes are able to find the antigen they need to bind to. There are three stages of differentiation within T cells and B cells. The first is the naïve cell (T cell or B cell), which are cells that don't yet have a specific antigen associated with it. The effector cells are actively destroying the pathogen and have an associated antigen with them. The memory cells aren't active but retain the "memory" of the past infection.

The process starts with antigen presentation. It's crucial that the cells recognize the self-cells and that they tell the difference between self- and non-self-antigens. Bacteria don't have self-antigens and are targeted for destruction. All cells express MHC molecules (except for erythrocytes). Some cells can present antigens along with their MHC molecules, including B cells, dendritic cells, and macrophages. These are known as professional APCs or antigen presenting cells. There are different types of T cells that have different capabilities of dealing with a pathogen or toxin.

Dendritic cells act by engulfing exogenous pathogens (toxins, parasites, or bacteria) and then travel to the lymph nodes, which are rich in T cells. The dendritic cells differentiate in transit so they can't phagocytize anything but can communicate with T cells. The antigen is cut in to smaller pieces and then gets displayed on the dendritic cell surface. In the lymph node, the antigen is coupled with an MCH that is recognized as a part of the self. Exogenous antigens are displayed along with MCH Class II molecules, which help activate T helper cells or CD4+ cells.

Endogenous antigens are made by either viruses or intracellular bacteria. The antigen presenting cell uses enzymes to digest proteins related to the pathogen, coupling them to the MCH and displaying the proteins on the cell surface. These are displayed with MHC class I molecules, activating the cytotoxic T cells (also called CD8+ cells). All cells except erythrocytes express the MCH class I proteins.

There are several names for CD8+ cells, including killer T cells and cytotoxic T lymphocytes. These have the ability to directly contribute to the death of infected, damaged, or dead cells. These cells are naïve at first and then bind to a MHC class I molecule, binding the T cell to the infected cell. The T cell becomes activated, undergoing clonal selection, forming a group of armed effector cells that then travel through the system looking for a matched MCH Class I plus antigen cell, which will be destroyed. The cytotoxic T lymphocyte releases granulysin and perforin, forming a pore in the target cell's plasma membrane, causing the cell to lyse. Granzyme is a protease that enters the damaged cell through the pores, resulting apoptosis (programmed cell death). This is a highly controlled process so it doesn't get out of control. When the infection is over with, the effector cells die off and are cleared away by phagocytes except for a select few that stay on as memory cells. They can reactivate to become effector cells when the antigen is present again.

CD4+ cells are also referred to as helper T cells or regulatory T cells. These are the mediators of the immune response, helping to maximize the adaptive immune system. They have no phagocytic or cytotoxic abilities but help manage the immune response. The express T cell receptors that recognize MHC Class II molecules, resulting in the release of cytokines, that influence the APC (antigen presenting cells). They provide extra signals that activate the CD8+ cells.

There are two types of helper cell responses that can be induced by a professional APC. These are called Th1 and Th2 responses. The Th1 response results in the release of interferon-gamma (that activates the macrophages and induces B cells to make antibodies leading to cell-mediated immunity). These are effective against intracellular pathogens. The Th2 response releases interleukin-5, inducing eosinophils to clear parasites. It also produces interleukin-4. The Th2 response is better for toxins, parasites, helminths, and extracellular bacteria. Most CD4+ cells die after the infection and are phagocytized (except for a few memory cells of the helper type).

There is more than one type of CD4+ cell. There are regulatory T cells that regulate and suppress the immune system, controlling responses to self-antigens (helping to control autoimmune diseases). Follicular helper T cells come from naïve T cells after being activated by antigens. They help B cells in humoral immunity because they are able to migrate B cells to the follicular parts of the lymphoid organs. Follicular helper cells also help increase immunological tolerance such that if they are abnormal, autoimmune diseases can occur.

B lymphocytes are the main antibody-producing cells in the blood plasma and are involved in humoral immunity. Antibodies made are Y-shaped proteins that are used to identify and neutralize foreign objects. There are five types of antibodies: IgA, IgD, IgE, IgG, and IgM—each of which has their own biological properties and handles different types of antigens.

There are five things that can happen to a binding of antigens and antibodies. There can be agglutination (a collection of infectious units), complement activation (increases inflammation and cell lysis), opsonization (coating the antigen to enhance phagocytosis), cell-mediated cytotoxicity, and neutralization (inhibiting adhesion of bacteria and viruses to mucosal cells).

B cells have their own unique B cell receptor, which is a membrane-bound antibody. Each B cell receptor recognizes and attaches only one specific antigen. B cells can recognize the antigen in their native form, while T cells recognize only processed antigens (connected to an MHC molecule). Once the B cell encounters the antigen, it differentiates further into a plasma cell, which is a B cell effector cell.

Plasma cells live about 2-3 days and secrete antibodies. The antibodies make antigens easier targets and trigger the complement cascade (leading to cell death). About 10 percent of cells go on to become memory B cells.

There are memory B cells and memory T cells. The body forms a database of B cells and T cells that recollect the antigen at a later time, controlling later infections through memory. This means that subsequent exposures to the antigen are faster and stronger than the initial response. This is what makes the response an "adaptive" response.

Passive memory is a short-lived response that lasts a few days or several months. Newborn infants receive maternal IgG antibodies across the placenta so they are immune to whatever the mother is immune to. Breast milk contains IgA antibodies that go to the gut of the baby so that they can protect the infant against GI infections.

Active memory is a long-term acquisition of immunity that can be acquired by an actual infection or artificially by immunization. Vaccines provide antigens that the body uses to make antibodies against a pathogen. The vaccine can be a live, attenuated virus or proteins that confer an immunological reaction. Viral vaccines tend to be live attenuated viruses, while bacterial vaccines are components of toxins or acellular parts of the microorganism that cannot cause disease but will confer immunity. Adjuvants are added to acellular vaccines to enhance the immune response.

Antigens can be anything that is large enough to be recognized by an immune cell. All proteins and many polysaccharides can become antigens. The part of the antigen that is interacting with the antibody is called the epitope (of which there can be many epitopes associated with a single antigen). Only a few cells of the immune system will respond to each antigen/epitope. There is the capability to make more than one trillion antibody molecules.

Immunity can be passive or active. It is active when the person makes their own antibodies against a pathogen or antigen. It is passive when antibodies are passed from one host individual to another. Both of these can be artificial or natural. Naturally-acquired active immunity is when a person gets sick with an illness and makes antibodies against the infectious organism. Naturally-acquired passive immunity involves the passage of antibodies from the placenta into the fetus or gets transferred through breast milk. Artificially-acquired active immunity is done by giving a person a vaccination. Artificially-acquired passive immunity is from the introduction of antibodies into a person (not a usual phenomenon).

Immunosuppression

Immunosuppression involves any type of reduction in the effectiveness of the immune system. Some parts of the immune system can be immunosuppressive to other parts of the immune system. Immunosuppression is deliberate when a person is given drugs to prevent organ transplant rejection, after a bone marrow transplant, or to treat autoimmune diseases. People can have immunosuppression and will be immunocompromised if they have chemotherapy or an HIV infection. This predisposes the person to getting various kinds of infectious diseases—both normal ones and opportunistic infections. The main thing that causes immunosuppression is the use of immunosuppressive drugs. Steroids were the first immunosuppressants identified, while things like azathioprine and cyclosporin are often used together to allow for an individual to have a less-well-matched transplant.

There are several diseases that can result in non-deliberate immunosuppression, such as certain cancer types, ataxia-telangiectasia, HIV disease, and complement deficiencies. These patients have an increase in opportunistic infections that they would not get if their immune system was normal. There are B cell and T cell deficiency states that a person can inherit from birth.

Key Takeaways

- The innate immune syndrome involves a nonspecific yet rapid response to a pathogen.
- There are barriers that protect the body from becoming infected.
- The cells of the innate immune system are mainly phagocytic cells.
- B cells and T cells make up the two main components of the adaptive immune system.

Quiz

1. What is the primary function of cytokines?
   a. To attach to pathogens to mark them for phagocytosis.
   b. To help cells in the phagocytic process.
   c. To attract immune cells to the site of infection.
   d. To suppress the immune response when it becomes hyperactive.

Answer: c. The main function of cytokines is to attract immune cells to the site of infection.

2. What is the major function of the complement cascade in the innate immune system?
   a. To attract neutrophils to the site of infection.
   b. To aid in eliminating dead cells and antibody-antigen complexes.
   c. To increase the release of inflammatory molecules.
   d. To bind to B cells that can then make antibodies.

Answer: b. Once activated, the compliment system helps the immune system eliminate dead cells and antibody-antigen complexes.

3. What activity is not considered a function of the innate immune system?
   a. Phagocytosis of pathogens
   b. Antigen-presentation
   c. Antibody production
   d. Chemotaxis of leukocytes

Answer: c. All of the above are considered functions of the innate immune system with the exception of antibody production, which is a function of the adaptive immune system.

4. Which cell in the immune system travels throughout the bloodstream and is attracted to the site of an infection or a breach in the barrier system?
   a. Macrophage
   b. Mast cell
   c. Neutrophil
   d. Histiocyte

Answer: c. It is the neutrophil that travels in the bloodstream, is attracted through chemotaxis to the site of an infection or breach in the barrier system, and kills invading microorganisms through phagocytosis.

5. Which cell type in the innate immune system is responsible for the release of histamine?
   a. Macrophage
   b. Mast cell
   c. Neutrophil
   d. Histiocyte

Answer: b. It is the mast cell that releases histamine as part of the allergic response, which is why the allergic response usually involves itching.

6. Which cells are the most efficient at the phagocytic process?
   a. Mast cells
   b. Eosinophils
   c. Histiocytes
   d. Macrophages

Answer: d. Macrophages are the cells that are most efficient in the phagocytic process.

7. Which type of cell in the adaptive immune system is a mature cell that has not yet encountered an antigen but which has the potential to become activated?
   a. CD4+ cell
   b. Effector T cell
   c. Naïve T cell
   d. Helper T cell

Answer: c. A naïve T cell has not yet become activated because it hasn't encountered an antigen.

8. Which type of cell in the adaptive immune system has the main function of providing the antigen that activates cytotoxicity in the adaptive immune system.
   a. Antigen-presenting cell
   b. CD8+ cell
   c. CD4+ cell
   d. Cytotoxic T cell

Answer: a. An antigen-presenting cell can be any kind of cell that presents an antigen to a naïve T cell, activating it as part of the adaptive immune system.

9. Which of the following cell type is not likely to be an antigen-presenting cell?
   a. Macrophage
   b. Histiocyte
   c. Dendritic cell
   d. B lymphocyte

Answer: b. Any of the above cell types can be antigen-presenting cells; however, histiocytes generally do not present antigens to T cells and have other functions in the immune system.

10. What is another term used to identify cytotoxic T cells?
    a. Helper T cells
    b. CD4+ cells
    c. Regulatory T cells
    d. CD8+ cells

Answer: d. Another name for cytotoxic T cells is CD8+ cells, because they express the CD8+ receptor glycoprotein on their cell surface.

Chapter 2: Common Bacterial Infections

Some common bacterial may arise spontaneously from a break in the protective barriers, such as the GI tract, respiratory tract, and skin. There are others that start as viral infections that turn into bacterial infections after the host is compromised by the initial infection. Bacteria are unicellular organisms, which are further described as either Gram-positive, Gram-negative, or Acid-Fast.

Cellulitis

Cellulitis is a bacterial infection of the skin, primarily the dermis and subcutaneous fat. Typical signs and symptoms include increasing redness, swelling, and warmth of the affected area. The borders of the redness are often diffuse and blanches when pressure is applied. Pain may be present as well. Lymphangitis involves the spread of cellulitis through the lymph tissues, which is the main complication of cellulitis. Fatigue and fever can be involved as well.

The face and legs are the most commonly affected sites of cellulitis, although a break in the skin anywhere can predispose a bacterial infection. Risk factors include leg swelling, obesity, diabetes, pregnancy, lymphedema, immunosuppression, and advanced age. Cellulitis of the face does not often require a break in the skin. The two most common infectious causes are Staphylococcus aureus and Group A Streptococcus. Besides lymphangitis, other complications of cellulitis include osteomyelitis and necrotizing fasciitis.

Predisposing conditions for cellulitis include insect bites, spider bites, animal bites, blisters, skin rashes, tattoos, eczema, athlete's foot, chickenpox blisters, injecting drugs, and recent surgery. Pregnancy, diabetes, and obesity affect circulation, leading to an increased risk of cellulitis. The diagnosis is mainly clinical, with the main differential diagnosis in leg infections being deep vein thrombosis.

The treatment for cellulitis involves antibiotics that should be given orally (although IVs might be necessary in severe cases). Common antibiotics include cloxacillin, amoxicillin, or cephalexin (with clindamycin and erythromycin used for penicillin-allergic patients). If MRSA is the confounding factor, then doxycycline or trimethoprim/sulfamethoxazole may be necessary. Staph infections can lead to abscess formation. The vast majority of patients get better within 7-10 days of treatment. The incidence of cellulitis is about 2 out of 1000 people per year. It is more common in patients living in dense populations with people sharing washing facilities with one another.

Rare complications of cellulitis include necrotizing fasciitis, which is also referred to as "flesh-eating bacteria"—a deeper infection that is a medical emergency, requiring high dose antibiotics and surgery to remove the infected tissue layers.

Bacterial Pneumonia

Bacterial pneumonia is a lower respiratory infection caused by a bacterial organism. Common symptoms include upper respiratory congestion (from a virus predating the infection), fever, chills, cough, chest pain, and dyspnea. Patients with a pneumococcal infection will have rusty sputum from hemoptysis.

The most common organism for all bacterial pneumonias except for neonates is Streptococcus pneumoniae. This is a Gram-positive organism. Other Gram-positive organisms that can cause pneumonia include Staphylococcus aureus and Bacillus anthracis.

Figure 3 shows a chest x-ray involved in bacterial pneumonia:

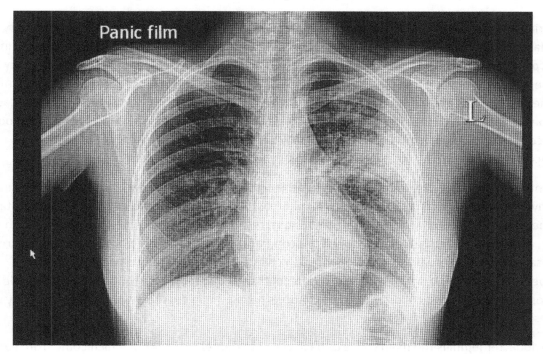

Figure 3

Gram-negative bacteria are less likely causes of pneumonia. Common Gram-negative causes of pneumonia include Escherichia coli, Klebsiella pneumoniae, Haemophilus influenzae, Moraxella catarrhalis, Bordetella pertussis, and Pseudomonas aeruginosa. These are organisms that actually originate in the GI tract and get into the lungs from inhalation of feces or vomit.

Atypical pneumonia stems from bacteria that have atypical or absent cell walls that don't take up the Gram staining in ways that are not similar to Gram-positive or Gram-negative bacteria. These include Legionella pneumophila, Mycoplasma pneumoniae, Chlamydophila pneumoniae, and Coxiella burnetii.

The bacteria in pneumonia enter the lungs through inhalation but it can come from the bloodstream if there are other body areas infected. The bacteria commonly live in the upper respiratory tract, continually being inhaled into the alveoli, but thwarted by the immune system. Normally, neutrophils will engulf the bacteria and prevent infection. However, they may also release cytokines that can increase the inflammatory response. The result is fever, fatigue, and chills. The fluid from the bloodstream, bacteria, and neutrophils can fill the alveoli, adversely affecting oxygen exchange. Bacteria can spread into the bloodstream, leading to bacteremia, sepsis, and septic shock.

The treatment of choice includes ventilatory support, oxygenation, and antibiotics. The choice of antibiotics depends on where the person lives. Amoxicillin and clarithromycin are the major antibiotics in the UK. In North America, there are more atypical infections, so that things like azithromycin, clarithromycin, and ciprofloxacin are drugs of choice. There are local variations in antibiotic resistances that should also be considered.

Bacterial Gastroenteritis

Bacterial gastroenteritis is also referred to as infectious diarrhea because diarrhea is the primary associated symptom. There is inflammation of the GI tract, particularly the stomach and small intestine. The typical symptoms are diarrhea, vomiting, and abdominal pain. Less commonly, patients may have fatigue, dehydration, and fever. The duration is less than 14 days. The most common cause of infectious diarrhea is rotavirus in children and norovirus in adults; however, the most common bacterial cause of gastroenteritis in adults is Campylobacter. Transmission can be from tainted water, infected foods, or close contact with an infected person. It is usually not necessary to test the stool as there is no appreciable treatment.

Preventative measures can be taken through drinking boiled or clean water, disposing of feces in a healthy way, washing with soap and water, and breastfeeding babies. Babies should get the rotavirus vaccine at two months of age. The main treatment, regardless of cause, is oral rehydration with salt, water, and sugar. IV fluids are necessary if the condition cannot be treated orally. Antibiotics are not necessary in most cases. Zinc is recommended in children. There are about two billion cases of gastroenteritis each year with about 1.3 million deaths (throughout the world). It affects people in developing countries and children the most. Adults have a small degree of immunity, especially with viruses.

Campylobacter jejuni is the main cause of bacterial gastroenteritis (most of which come from eating tainted poultry). Bacteria cause about 15 percent of cases of infection in children. Other causes include Escherichia coli, Shigella, and Salmonella. Bacteria multiply in warm food that is contaminated, creating enough bacteria to cause infection. Typical foods related to bacterial gastroenteritis include raw meat, poultry, seafood, eggs, unpasteurized milk, raw sprouts, vegetable and fruit juices, and unpasteurized soft cheeses. Cholera (an infection of the small intestine caused by Vibrio cholerae) is a common cause of gastroenteritis in the developing world, secondary to consuming tainted food and water.

Clostridium difficile causes disease because of toxin production. It is a cause of diarrhea that is more common in older individuals. Infants may have no symptoms yet still be carriers of the disease. It is mainly caused by taking antibiotics that destroy normal body flora. Staphylococcus aureus infection can always occur when antibiotics are taken. Acute traveler's diarrhea is often bacterial, while chronic disease is often from parasites. There is an increased risk in people who take proton pump inhibitors and Histamine-2 blockers.

Peritonitis

Peritonitis is any inflammation of the peritoneum, which is the thin layer of tissue that lines the GI tract and the inside of the abdominal wall. Typical symptoms include abdominal distention, severe abdominal pain, fever, and weight loss.   It is usually caused by a perforation of the GI tract or from appendicitis. It may be generalized in the abdomen or localized.

Typical findings besides abdominal pain include abdominal tenderness, rebound tenderness (a positive Blumberg sign), and guarding. Rebound tenderness is somewhat specific to peritonitis; however, rigidity is the most specific finding seen in the disease. The pain and tenderness can be localized or generalized. The pain commonly starts as generalized pain, and becomes more localized as the parietal peritoneum becomes involved.

Besides the above listed abdominal symptoms, patients will have fever, ileus (intestinal paralysis), nausea, vomiting, sinus tachycardia, and bloating. Ileus will show up as silent bowel sounds. There will be a leakage of fluid into the peritoneal space with decreased central venous pressure, shock, acute renal insufficiency, electrolyte disturbances, peritoneal abscesses, septicemia, and organ failure.

The most common cause of peritonitis is a perforation of some part of the GI tract. The distal esophagus can be perforated from Boerhaave syndrome, the stomach can be perforated, and any other part of the GI tract can be perforated. It can be from diverticulitis, appendicitis, inflammatory bowel disease, intestinal infarction, cholecystitis, colorectal cancer, or abdominal trauma. Mixed organisms are at fault, particularly Escherichia coli, Bacteroides fragilis, and other Gram-negative and anaerobic bacterial species.

Disruption of the peritoneum can happen without perforation of a hollow viscus seen in trauma, surgery, peritoneal dialysis, and intraperitoneal chemotherapy, with the most common species being coagulase negative Staphylococcus and Staphylococcus aureus (as well as Candida and fungi). Spontaneous bacterial peritonitis stems from an infection without an obvious source. It can occur in patients who have ascites and in children. Tuberculosis can affect the peritoneum and can cause peritonitis. Pelvic inflammatory disease from an STD can lead to peritonitis.

The major risk factors for peritonitis include alcoholism, previous peritonitis, liver disease, pelvic inflammatory disease, poor immune system, and ascites. The main treatment of peritonitis include surgery to remove abscesses and antibiotic therapy.

Sinusitis

Sinusitis or "rhinosinusitis" is an inflammation and infection of the sinuses. Typical symptoms include thick nasal drainage, facial pain, and nasal congestion. Severe cases include a lack of smell, sore throat, cough, fever, and headaches. The cough tends to be nocturnal. It is rarely complicated. It is referred as acute if it lasts less than 4 weeks and chronic when it lasts longer than 3 months (12 weeks).

Figure 4 describes the pathology seen in sinusitis:

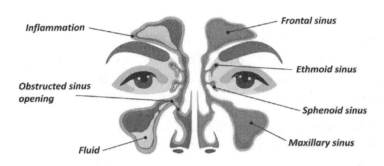

Figure 4

There are four classifications of sinusitis. The first is acute sinusitis that lasts up to four weeks. Recurrent sinusitis involves having four or more episodes of acute sinusitis per year. Subacute sinusitis lasts from four weeks to twelve weeks. Chronic sinusitis lasts longer than twelve weeks. These are otherwise similar in symptoms and differ only in length of time the symptoms last.

The classic symptoms include having a headache or facial pain over the affected sinus or sinuses. The pain is worse when lying down or bending over. There is thick nasal discharge that is green or yellow in color and may be malodorous. A toothache or localized headache can be present. The infection can spread to the eye socket with may affect the patients sight. Osteomyelitis of the bones can be a complicating factor. Chronic sinusitis is often complicated by post-nasal drip. Halitosis can be a typical sign. Sinus headaches may mimic migraine headaches, and be misdiagnosed.

While many cases of sinusitis are bacterial, it can be caused by allergies, nasal structural problems, or air pollution. Most are viral but those lasting longer than 10 days are likely to be bacterial, especially if the person gets worse after improving. People with poor immunity, cystic fibrosis, and asthma will have recurrent disease. X-rays do not help; however, direct visualization or CT scan of the sinuses are necessary if the patient does not recover quickly.

The treatment of acute sinusitis of any cause is watchful waiting unless the symptoms are present for longer than 7-10 days or get worse. The first line agents include amoxicillin or amoxicillin/clavulanate. Rarely patients will require surgery. About 10-30 percent of individuals in the Northern Hemisphere will get a case of acute sinusitis with 12 percent experiencing an episode of chronic sinusitis at some point.

Acute Otitis Media

Otitis media involves a middle ear infection. It can be just acute otitis media (AOM) or otitis media with effusion (OME). The pain of acute otitis media is of sudden onset, particularly seen in young children. It involves poor eating habits and fever, with babies pulling on their ear. OME, on the other hand has no symptoms except for a feeling of ear fullness. Chronic suppurative otitis media is a chronic infection of two weeks or longer that results in discharge from the ear. It can be a complication of AOM. It is rarely painful. All types of otitis media can be linked to hearing loss. In OME, the patient may have chronic hearing loss. Risk factors include using pacifiers, being exposed to smoke, and attending daycare. Children with down syndrome are at a higher risk of OME.

Figure 5 shows what otitis media looks like anatomically:

OTITIS MEDIA

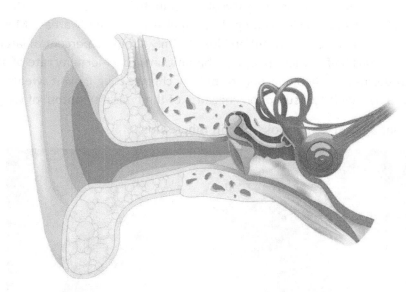

Figure 5

The main symptom is ear pain but other symptoms can be irritability and fever. Usually, other respiratory symptoms can be present as it ultimately stems from an upper respiratory infection. Ear discharge is seen with perforation of the tympanic membrane or with otitis externa. The main cause of the problem is Eustachian tube dysfunction, causing buildup of fluid in the middle ear cavity. It is purely a clinical diagnosis, with visualization of the tympanic membrane showing the redness and bulging of the membrane. Severe cases that do not resolve require a CT scan of the temporal bone, MRI scan of the ear, or a tympanogram.

The most common bacterial organisms associated with acute otitis media include Streptococcus pneumoniae, Haemophilus influenzae, Moraxella catarrhalis, and Staphylococcus aureus. These are usually secondary infections that start out as virally-oriented infections.

There are things that decrease the risk of otitis media, including pneumococcus vaccination, influenza vaccination, early breastfeeding, and avoiding tobacco exposure. Pain medications can be used in cases where the pain is present. Antibiotics should be reserved for those under aged 2 or with severe disease. The antibiotic used as a first-line agent is amoxicillin. Frequent cases can be managed with tympanostomy tubes. Antibiotics can be used in cases of effusion to clear out the effusion sooner (but there are side effects of taking antibiotics).

Acute otitis media affects about 11 percent of people per year. About 50 percent of cases occur in children under 5 years of age and it is more common in boys. Only about 5 percent of cases will be chronic in nature. It affects up to 80 percent of kids prior to age 10 years. Very rarely, deaths can occur from this disorder (with only about 3000-5000 deaths per year worldwide). Complications include mastoiditis, subperiosteal abscess, bony destruction of nearby bone, meningitis, and venous thrombosis.

Tuberculosis

Tuberculosis is a bacterial infection caused by Mycobacterium tuberculosis, an acid-fast bacterial species. Its main location of infection is the lungs but can affect other body areas. Most patients have no symptoms, which is considered "latent tuberculosis". Only about 10 percent of latent infections lead to active disease, which kills half of these people. (This amounts to a mortality rate of about 5 percent). Typical signs and symptoms include blood-tinged sputum, chronic cough, night sweats, fever, and weight loss. It used to be called "consumption" because of the typical symptom of weight loss.

Figure 6 depicts what a chest x-ray looks like in tuberculosis:

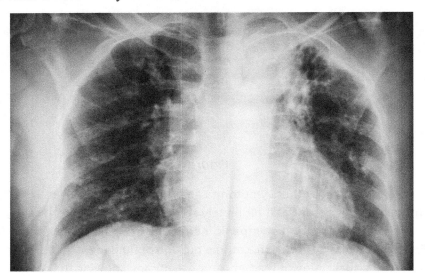

Figure 6

Extrapulmonary disease occurs in up to 20 percent of cases, seen more commonly in immunosuppressed individuals and young people. Extrapulmonary sites of TB include the lung pleura, the CNS (meningitis), lymphatic system, bones and joints, and the genitourinary system. The most common extrapulmonary site is the lymph nodes, which will be seen as a painless, enlarging lymph node. A more serious form of TB includes disseminated tuberculosis or miliary tuberculosis, in which the disease is everywhere. This accounts for 10 percent of extrapulmonary TB.

Tuberculosis is spread in the air when a tuberculous patient coughs, sneezes, or spits. It is more commonly seen in smokers and HIV patients. The diagnosis of active disease is seen in the chest x-ray, TB test, and sputum evaluation. The only way to prevent the disease is screening high risk patients, early treatment of active cases, and using the BCG (bacillus Calmette Guerin) vaccine. Multiple antibiotics are necessary because of an increasing rate of multiple drug resistance. New infections affect about 1 percent of patients per year with about a third of all people in the world being infected. About 95 percent of cases are seen in developing countries. In African and Asian countries, 80 percent of people will have a positive TB test, while in the US, about 5-10 percent of people will have a positive skin test.

Osteomyelitis

Osteomyelitis or OM is a bacterial infection of bone (but can rarely be fungal). The typical symptoms include fever, overlying redness, fatigue, and weakness. The long bones are mainly affected in children, while the hips, spine, and feet are the most common sites in adults. The infection can be hematogenous or from local infection. Typical risk factors for osteomyelitis include undergoing a splenectomy, local trauma, IV drug use, and diabetes. It is symptomatically diagnosed with x-rays, bone biopsy, and blood cultures.

Figure 7 shows the pathophysiology of osteomyelitis:

OSTEOMYELITIS

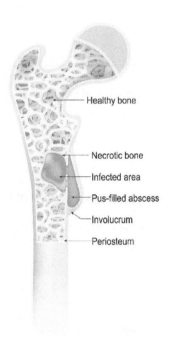

Figure 7

The causes of osteomyelitis are somewhat dependent on the person's age. Newborns tend to get Streptococcus, Enterobacter, and Staphylococcus infections. Young children can get Staphylococcus, Streptococcus, Haemophilus, and Enterobacter infections. Adults can get Staphylococcus, Enterobacter, or Streptococcus infections. Sickle cell anemia patients can get Salmonella infections.

Adults tend to get the disease from being debilitated, having IV drug use, infected root canals, or being on immunosuppressive drugs. Osteomyelitis occurs in up to 3 percent of patients with tuberculosis. All forms of osteomyelitis have Staphylococcus aureus as the primary cause in most cases, regardless of age. Exposed bone from a traumatic injury is a common reason to get osteomyelitis. Besides Staphylococcus aureus, other causes of a bone infection can be Escherichia coli, Pseudomonas aeruginosa, and Serratia marcescens. Less commonly, fungal infections can be bony in nature. The two most common fungal species include Blastomyces dermatitidis and Coccidioides immitis.

Treatment involves surgery to remove dead and infected tissues, and antibiotics. Amputation may be necessary if there is inadequate blood flow. The incidence is about 2 out of 100,000 people affected per year. It affects primarily young people and old people; it carries a high risk of mortality without antibiotics and surgery.

Key Takeaways

- Bacterial infections may be caused by Gram-positive, Gram-negative, or Acid-fast organisms.
- Cellulitis generally stems from a Streptococcus or Staphylococcus infection.
- The most common cause of bacterial pneumonia is Streptococcus pneumoniae.
- The risk of morbidity and mortality from bacterial infections has decreased since the time of antibiotics.

Quiz

1. What is the main complication of bacterial cellulitis?
   a. Sepsis
   b. Lymphangitis
   c. Osteomyelitis
   d. Compartment syndrome

Answer: b. Lymphangitis is the most common complication of bacterial cellulitis.

2. What bacterial organism is the most likely cause of cellulitis?
   a. Staphylococcus aureus
   b. Klebsiella pneumoniae
   c. Escherichia coli
   d. Peptostreptococcus

Answer: a. Staphylococcus aureus is a major cause of cellulitis. The others are not causes of cellulitis.

3. Which part of the body might be most affected by cellulitis without a break in the skin?
   a. Chest
   b. Buttocks
   c. Face
   d. Hand

Answer: c. Both the face and the legs are most likely to be affected by cellulitis. The face rarely stems from a break in the skin.

4. What defines a type of pneumonia that is said to be atypical?

a. The organism reacts atypically to antibiotics

b. The symptoms are not typical of other types of pneumonia

c. The organism has an absent or atypical cell wall

d. The organism follows an atypical course of action

Answer: c. The organism causing an atypical pneumonia is atypical because it has an unusual cell wall that doesn't pick up Gram stain dye the same way as Gram-positive or Gram-negative organisms do.

5. What organism is a cause of atypical pneumonia?
   a. Mycoplasma pneumoniae
   b. Pseudomonas aeruginosa
   c. Klebsiella pneumoniae
   d. Moraxella catarrhalis

Answer: a. Mycoplasma pneumoniae is a common cause of atypical pneumonia.

6. What is not considered a drug of choice for bacterial pneumonia in North America?
   a. Azithromycin
   b. Clarithromycin
   c. Ciprofloxacin
   d. Penicillin

Answer: d. Penicillin resistance is very high in North America so penicillin wouldn't be the drug of choice for bacterial pneumonia. The others are considered first-line agents for this type of pneumonia.

7. What is the main source of an infection with Campylobacter?
   a. Raw poultry
   b. Vegetables
   c. Tainted water
   d. Raw seafood

Answer: a. The main source of Campylobacter is eating raw poultry.

8. What is the main cause of cholera in developing countries?
   a. Escherichia
   b. Vibrio
   c. Shigella
   d. Clostridium

Answer: b. Vibrio cholerae is the main cause of cholera in developing countries.

9. What is the main cause of Clostridium difficile gastroenteritis?
   a. Tainted water
   b. Uncooked eggs
   c. Antibiotic use
   d. Unwashed fruit

Answer: c. Clostridium difficile gastroenteritis is mainly caused by taking antibiotics that kill the normal, protective gut flora, allowing Clostridium to proliferate.

10. What is the most common bacterial organism seen in cases of osteomyelitis?
    a. Mycobacterium tuberculosis
    b. Enterobacter species
    c. Salmonella
    d. Staphylococcus aureus

Answer: d. Regardless of age, the most common cause of osteomyelitis is Staphylococcus aureus.

Chapter 3: Common Viral Infections

For the most part, viral infections are more common than bacterial infections. While there are antiviral treatments for some types of viral infections, many resolve spontaneously as patient's own immune system eliminates the infection. Infections with viruses can by systemic or localized to a certain body area, such as the respiratory tract, liver, or gastrointestinal tract.

Influenza

Influenza is primarily a respiratory infection that also has non-respiratory symptoms. Typical symptoms include fever, nasal congestion, myalgias, sore throat, coughing, headache, and fatigue. The incubation period is two days and the length of the illness is about a week to two weeks. Children may have nausea and vomiting, which isn't seen in adults. The main complications of influenza include viral pneumonia, bacterial pneumonia, sinus infection, worsening of asthma, and worsening of heart failure.

The viral types of influenza are type A, type B, and type C. These viruses are spread through the air through coughing or sneezing. It can also be spread through touching contaminated surfaces and then touching the eyes. The infection can be passed before, during, and after a clinical infection. There are rapid tests of the sputum or nose that can be done but they have a high false negative rate. The polymerase chain reaction (detecting RNA in the viral genome) is highly accurate.

The three ways to avoid an infection include frequent handwashing, wearing a surgical mask, and getting a vaccination every year. The vaccine generally protects the person against 3-4 types of influenza viruses. Antiviral drugs are available to treat influenza but are only helpful when given within the first day or so after onset of symptoms.

There are 3-5 million cases of influenza annually with about 500,000 deaths per year (throughout the world). Outbreaks tend to occur in the winter months (except near the equator) with most deaths in the young, those with health problems, and old patients. Pandemics occur less frequently. The influenza pandemics include the Spanish flu (1918), Asian flu (1957), Hong Kong flu (1968) and H1N1 flu (2009).

The influenza vaccine is perhaps the best way to prevent the disease. It is recommended for all immunocompromised people, those with chronic diseases (heart disease, diabetes, and asthma), children, and the elderly. The vaccine reduces the incidence of influenza and decreases COPD exacerbations. It decreases the rate of infection in HIV patients, cancer patients, and organ transplant patients. Because of the mutation rate of influenza, the vaccine is successful for only a few years. The vaccine is based on which viruses are more likely to cause infection in any given year. The vaccine takes two weeks to become effective against the flu. The shot can lead to flu symptoms as a side effect of the vaccine.

There are two antiviral drugs (amantadine and rimantadine) that block the replication of the influenza A virus, being viral ion channel blockers. They are effective against influenza A but don't work against influenza B (which don't have the same ion channel). The resistance to the drugs is high, in part because they are available over the counter in several countries. For this reason, these drugs are not necessarily recommended for use against influenza.

Upper Respiratory Infection

An upper respiratory infection or URI is any illness that infects the upper respiratory tract, including the larynx, pharynx, sinuses, and nose. While other organisms can cause these types of infections, viruses cause the vast majority of infections. There are billions of cases of URIs per year (about 17 billion), with only about 3000 deaths annually from the virus throughout the year.

URIs can be classified by the area of the body that was inflamed. Rhinitis is an infection of the nasal mucosa; rhinosinusitis is an infection of the nose and sinuses; nasopharyngitis is an infection of the nose and throat; pharyngitis infects the pharynx and tonsils; laryngitis infects the larynx; laryngotracheitis is in the larynx and trachea. The length of time of symptoms is about 14 days. In most cases, when the disease is rhinitis, pharyngitis, and laryngitis, it is referred to as the common cold. If the illness is sinusitis, ear infection or bronchitis, it is said to be a complication of the common cold. The incubation period is about 1-3 days. The change of mucus from clear to opaque and green is a natural part of the infection. In general, antibiotics are not recommended for an uncomplicated URI.

The upper respiratory infection causes disease by activating the immune response rather than by damaging the cells. The viruses cause changes in the tight junctions between the epithelial cells of the upper respiratory tract. This allows the virus to get into the tissues beneath the epithelium, causing both an innate immune system response and an adaptive immune system response. More than 200 viruses cause URIs, but the most common is the rhinovirus, which is thought to be responsible for at least half of all URIs. Other viruses that can cause URIs include coronavirus, respiratory syncytial virus, influenza and parainfluenza.

Respiratory Syncytial Virus

The human respiratory syncytial virus or RSV is a virus that primarily causes respiratory tract infections. It is especially found in infants and early childhood, where it causes lower respiratory tract infections. Prophylactic medication (palivizumab) can be used in preterm infants or infants who have bronchopulmonary dysplasia and congenital heart defects. Treatment is often supportive, including oxygen therapy, fever control, and CPAP in some cases. It is more common in the winter months or in the rainy season in tropical parts of the world.

Figure 8 depicts the respiratory syntytial virus:

Respiratory Syncytial Virus

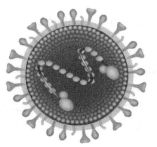

Figure 8

The incidence is extremely high with 60 percent of babies becoming infected in the first year of life and about 100 percent of children infected by the age of 2 years. About 2-3 percent will have bronchiolitis, which generally requires hospitalization. The protective immunity that comes with the infection does not last forever so people can get the infection at an older age. This means that even older individuals can get a severe case of RSV infection.

The incubation period is 4-5 days. It is exactly like the common cold in adults but can cause bronchiolitis and pneumonia in kids under one year of age. It rarely can cause death in infancy. The symptoms of cough, congestion, listlessness, fever, and poor appetite are common in infants and young children with RSV. Recurrent wheezing can occur in infants with RSV. Pneumonia is especially common in patients who are immunosuppressed (such as transplant patients). It can be tested for by doing a polymerase chain reaction (PCR) test in the blood sample.

The infection itself will last from 2-8 days in normal children but symptoms can last for up to 3 weeks. Typical complications of RSV include pneumonia, bronchiolitis, otitis media, and secondary bacterial infections.

Viral Gastroenteritis

Viral gastroenteritis is any infection and subsequent inflammation of the stomach, the small intestine, and the colon. There are several viruses that cause of gastroenteritis. In adults, the most common virus is the norovirus, while in children, the most common virus is the rotavirus. Adenovirus and astrovirus also known to cause viral gastroenteritis. Rotavirus in children happens at a similar rate in both the developed and developing parts of the world. Viruses make up about 70 percent of cases of infectious diarrhea in children.

The main symptoms of viral gastroenteritis are watery diarrhea, nausea, and vomiting. Less common symptoms include fever, chills, headache, and abdominal pain. The incubation period is 12-24 hours, with symptoms lasting 1-3 days (but can last longer). The most common complication is dehydration, when more fluids are lost through diarrhea and vomiting than are gained through drinking. People who are very young, very old, or immunosuppressed have an increased likelihood of getting dehydration. Severe dehydration can result in IV fluids.

The virus is transmitted through the fecal oral route or by touching contaminated surfaces. It can become airborne if the person vomits. Washing hands can reduce the transmission of the disease. Sharing eating utensils can transmit the virus. Norovirus can live on multiple surfaces that aren't washed with bleach. People without symptoms are able to transmit the virus. Even after full recovery, a previously infected person can transmit the virus for up to two weeks.

Outbreaks tend to happen when people are living or working in close quarters. Stool can be cultured for the virus but this is rarely necessary. Antibiotics don't help but things like bismuth subsalicylate and loperamide can be used in adults (but not in children). The main treatment is to use oral rehydration to prevent dehydration. Children are more likely to become dehydrated because of their small size. Oral rehydration solutions and a BRAT diet can help in the recovery (bananas, rice cereal, applesauce, and toast).

Viral Hepatitis

Viral hepatitis is an infection that causes inflammation of the liver. It can be an acute infection or a chronic infection. There are generally five different viruses that cause hepatitis that are actually unrelated to one another. These include hepatitis A, hepatitis B, hepatitis C, hepatitis D, and hepatitis E. Hepatitis A and E are transmitted by the fecal-oral route, while hepatitis B, C, and D are transmitted via blood and body fluids. Minor viruses that can cause hepatic inflammation include Epstein-Barr virus, yellow fever, and cytomegalovirus. Extremely rare cases of herpes virus hepatitis have been uncovered.

The incubation period for the types of hepatitis is wide. It is as short as 15 days and as long as 160 days (for hepatitis B). In hepatitis B, about 5-10 percent become chronic, while with hepatitis C, about 70 percent will become chronic. There is a vaccine for hepatitis A that lasts 10 years and a 3-shot injection vaccine for hepatitis B that offers lifetime protection.

Hepatitis A is a picornavirus transmitted by contaminated food or water. It only causes acute hepatitis and, after one episode, the person is immune from future infections with the virus. It is excreted in the feces two weeks after contracting the virus and will remain in the feces for a week after jaundice starts. The incubation period is an average of 28 days. Most people recover within two months; however, 15 percent of people will have ongoing symptoms for 6-12 months.

Hepatitis B is caused by a hepadnavirus that can result in acute or chronic infection. About 15 percent of people will develop a chronic infection. It is passed through sexual intercourse, dirty needles, unsanitary tattoos, blood transfusion, breastfeeding, and through the placenta. Half the time, the source is never discovered. Complications of chronic disease include cirrhosis and hepatocellular carcinoma. There are drugs that can help treat chronic infections that work in about 65 percent of patients.

Hepatitis C is a Flaviviridae virus that is transmitted through blood or body fluids, including sexual activity. It can cross the placenta. It leads to cirrhosis and hepatocellular cancer in some cases. It is often asymptomatic for a long period of time but can develop severe disease if they also get hepatitis A or hepatitis B. A combination of ribavirin and interferon can improve chronic hepatitis. It is the most common chronic blood infection in the US.

Hepatitis D comes from the Deltavirus subtype and is similar to a viroid because it can only grow if the person is also infected the hepatitis B virus. It is a defective virus that cannot exist independently and is passed through blood and body fluids.

Hepatitis E is a Hepeviridae strain of hepatitis that is similar to hepatitis A. It is passed through fecal oral route and there isn't a vaccine for the virus. It is generally mild except for women in the third trimester of pregnancy where it can be fatal. It is seen more often in areas in and around India.

Epstein-Barr Viral Infections (EBV)

Epstein-Barr viruses are Herpesviruses can cause several diseases, including infectious mononucleosis. The disease is seen most often in developing countries, where the patient generally gets the infection by the time they are 18 months of age. Adults give it to children when they pre-chew the child's food. In the US, about half of all children aged 5 years will be positive for the antibody.

The Epstein-Barr virus is highly linked to Burkitt's lymphoma and nasopharyngeal cancer. It is believed also to cause several autoimmune diseases, multiple sclerosis, and chronic fatigue syndrome. It is also associated with other forms of cancer, such as Hodgkin's lymphoma, gastric cancer, and malignant conditions associated with HIV disease, such as hairy leukoplakia and central nervous system lymphomas. Burkitt's lymphoma is a kind of non-Hodgkin's lymphoma seen mostly in Africa near the Equator. The virus is linked to lymphoma only when the patient also has an infection with malaria. It forms a jaw-related tumor that can be treated with cyclophosphamide as a form of chemotherapy. Nasopharyngeal cancer and EBV is found in the southern parts of China and in Africa.

The symptoms of an infection with EBV include sore throat, fever, swollen lymph glands, hepatomegaly, and splenomegaly. Rarely, CNS and heart problems can develop. It is not particularly dangerous in pregnancy but the infection lasts 1-2 months. It remains dormant in the blood and throat for the duration of the patient's life but can reactivate periodically and infect others. It can be passed in utero and a person can become sick with the virus even though the person is already seropositive. Transmission only comes from contact with infected saliva and not through any other means (blood, stool, or airborne).

There is no specific treatment for EBV-related infectious mononucleosis other than managing the symptoms. Severe cases can be treated with corticosteroids to decrease the inflammatory response. There is no vaccine for the infection and no antiviral agents that can improve the outcome of the disease process. The infection runs its course in about 2-4 months.

Key Takeaways

- Viral infections can infect the entire person or can be organ-specific, such as in hepatitis or gastroenteritis.
- Respiratory infections include RSV infections, any of the cold viruses, or the influenza virus.
- Gastroenteritis is viral about 70 percent of the time and leads to vomiting and watery diarrhea.
- There are five major types of hepatitis that can be transmitted via the fecal-oral route of via the blood and body fluids.

Quiz

1. What is the incubation period of the influenza virus (the time between exposure and clinical illness)?
   a. 2 days
   b. 5 days
   c. 8 days
   d. 14 days

Answer: a. The patient can get sick within two days of being exposed to the influenza virus.

2. What symptom of influenza is often seen in children but is not seen in adults with the disease?
   a. Fever
   b. Nasal congestion

c. Myalgias

d. Vomiting

Answer: d. Nausea and vomiting are two symptoms seen in children with influenza but aren't seen in adults with the virus.

3. Which influenza pandemic occurred during the winter of 1918?
    a. Asian flu
    b. Spanish flu
    c. Hong Kong flu
    d. H1N1 flu

Answer: b. The Spanish flu pandemic killed about 50 million people in 1918.

4. When should antibiotics be given in an upper respiratory infection?
    a. If there is a fever of greater than 100 degrees for 24 hours or more
    b. If the mucus becomes green in color
    c. It shouldn't be given in a URI
    d. It should be given if there is tonsillitis

Answer: c. In general, there is no indication to give antibiotics for an uncomplicated upper respiratory infection.

5. What type of virus strain is most likely to cause an upper respiratory infection?
    a. Respiratory syncytial virus
    b. Rhinovirus
    c. Adenovirus
    d. Coronavirus

Answer: b. When it comes to upper respiratory infections, the most common viral type is the rhinovirus. The others are less likely to cause a URI.

6. Approximately what percentage of children will be infected with respiratory syncytial virus in the first two years of life?
    a. 30 percent
    b. 50 percent
    c. 75 percent
    d. 100 percent

Answer: d. Virtually all children will have an RSV infection sometime in the first two years of life.

7. What is the incubation period for viral gastroenteritis?
    a. 12-24 hours
    b. 2-4 days
    c. 5-7 days
    d. 7-10 days

Answer: a. The incubation period for viral gastroenteritis is 12-24 hours, but can be as long as 1 day after becoming infected.

8. What virus is most likely to cause viral gastroenteritis in adult patients?
   a. Astrovirus
   b. Rotavirus
   c. Norovirus
   d. Adenovirus

Answer: c. The most common cause of viral gastroenteritis in adults is the norovirus. This is not the case in children, who get more rotavirus infections.

9. Besides oral rehydration, what can be given to an adult to help prevent dehydration in cases of viral gastroenteritis?
   a. Tincture of opium
   b. Mylanta
   c. Calcium carbonate
   d. Loperamide

Answer: d. Loperamide can be obtained without a prescription and very successful in managing the diarrhea seen in viral gastroenteritis.

10. Which type of cancer is not linked to an infection with the Epstein-Barr virus?
    a. Burkitt's lymphoma
    b. Hepatocellular carcinoma
    c. Gastric cancer
    d. Nasopharyngeal cancer

Answer: b. The Epstein-Barr virus is associated with all of the above types of cancer except for hepatocellular carcinoma, which is not connected to EBV.

Chapter 4: Common Fungal Infections

Fungal infections range from minor to more severe diseases requiring aggressive therapy. Fungal organisms are not significantly different, biochemically, from human cells so they tend to be more difficult to kill without causing significant side effects. Common fungal infections include Aspergillosis, Candidiasis, Histoplasmosis, Cryptococcosis and Coccidiomycosis.

Systemic Candidiasis

While candidiasis can be benign, this chapter discusses a more serious type of candidiasis, called systemic candidiasis. This is a serious infection of various parts of the body, including the bones, the eyes, the heart, the brain, and the blood. There are more than two hundred kinds of Candida; however, only five species are responsible for 90 percent of systemic infections. The most common place where systemic candidiasis is found is in the bloodstream. This is referred to as candidemia and causes fever and chills.

Figure 9 shows what oral candidiasis looks like. Certain patients can ultimately develop systemic disease from this type of infection:

ORAL CANDIDIASIS

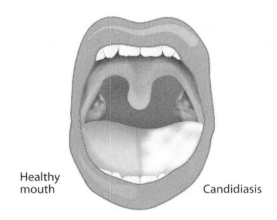

Healthy mouth   Candidiasis

Figure 9

Systemic candidiasis is the most common fungal infection in patients who are hospitalized in developed countries. Candida may be difficult to diagnose at it will not always grow out of the bloodstream. The infection can be so severe that the patient has shock—with decreased blood pressure, tachypnea, and tachycardia. Other parts of the body that can be affected are the abdomen, brain and spinal cord, eyes, spleen, joints, muscles, bones, liver, kidneys, and heart. There are different symptoms depending on what part of the body is affected. When the eyes are affected, there is blurry vision and photophobia. When the heart is affected, there is endocarditis with petechiae, weight loss, peripheral edema, dyspnea, and fever. These patients are extremely sick and may have confusing symptoms that mimic other disorders.

The cause of candidiasis is the species Candida—primarily the following five species: C. krusei, C. tropicalis, C. parapsilosis, C. glabrata, and C. albicans (with C. albicans being the most common species identified). While Candida is commonly found in the normal skin and GI tract, it can overgrow in the bloodstream. From there, it can settle in any one of the other body areas mentioned.

Things that increase the risk of systemic disease include people how are immunosuppressed, those who are in an ICU, people who've had GI surgery, patients with a central venous catheter, premature infants, diabetics, people in renal failure, people on broad-spectrum antibiotics, and people with neutropenia.

When symptoms develop, the diagnosis should be suspected in patients at high risk and can be confirmed by a blood culture or culture of the CSF for fungal organisms. The blood culture will be negative half the time so further testing of specific organs with an MRI may be necessary. The recommended treatment is IV antifungal medications, including echinocandin, or a combination of fluconazole and amphotericin B. In some cases, prophylactic antifungal medication can prevent disease.

The prognosis of patients with systemic candidiasis depends on patient factors and the location of the infection. These patients are often already very sick so it is hard to say if they die from an underlying problem or from candidiasis. The mortality rate for candidemia is about 20-30 percent, even with treatment.

Aspergillosis

Aspergillosis involves any one of several diseases caused by Aspergillus, a type of fungus. It tends to occur in patients who have certain underlying diseases, such as pulmonary tuberculosis or COPD (but who are not necessarily immunosuppressed). The different kinds of aspergillosis include an aspergilloma, chronic pulmonary aspergillosis, and allergic bronchopulmonary aspergillosis. The different types can be related to one another.

Figure 10 indicates an aspergilloma of the lung and what the fungal particle looks like:

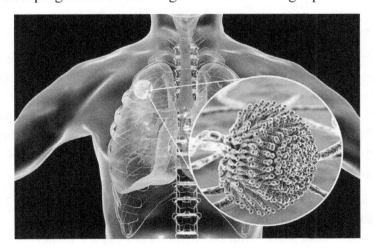

Figure 10

Chronic pulmonary aspergillosis is a long-standing aspergillus infection of the lung. Aspergillus fumigatus is almost always the species responsible for this illness. An aspergilloma, also known as a fungus ball, is a clump of mold which exists in a body cavity such as a paranasal sinus or the lung. Allergic bronchopulmonary aspergillosis is a condition involving an exaggerated response of the immune system to the fungus Aspergillus (most commonly Aspergillus fumigatus). It commonly develops in patients with asthma or cystic fibrosis. Less common places to find aspergillus is the eye, nailbed, sinuses, and ear canal.

Disseminated aspergillosis involves patients who are immunosuppressed because of leukemia, HIV disease, chemotherapy or a stem cell transplant. Spores get into the lungs and then spread to the bloodstream, where the body has no immune response. The major organs become involved, such as the kidneys and the heart valves. People inhale the spores every day but the immune system fights off an active infection.

There may be no symptoms of an aspergilloma so that it is found incidentally. It can cause massive pulmonary bleeding, hemoptysis, and chest pain. The infection can be systemic in the lungs, leading to fever, chest pain, dyspnea, and cough. If it isn't controlled, it spreads to the bloodstream, leading to symptoms of shock, delirium, blood clots, and seizures. Liver and kidney failure often are precursors to death.

Pulmonary aspergillosis can be seen as classic findings on a CT of the chest or even a chest x-ray. A biopsy stained with silver stain will show up the cell walls of the fungus and the budding hyphae. They have specific branching of the hyphae which can reliably diagnose the disease. The best way to make the diagnosis is through a biopsy of infected tissue. There are no blood tests or cultures that can identify the disorder.

The major treatments for aspergillosis include surgical debridement, voriconazole, and liposomal amphotericin B. Steroids can suppress allergic bronchopulmonary aspergillosis for 6-9 months. Itraconazole can be given along with steroids to decrease the dose of steroids necessary to blunt the immune response. The biggest problem with drugs like itraconazole is that there are a lot of drug resistances, especially with Aspergillus fumigatus.

Histoplasmosis

Histoplasmosis goes by many names including "caver's disease", "reticuloendotheliosis", "Cave disease", "spelunker's lung", and "Darling's disease". It primarily leads to lung disease but can be disseminated. It may be fatal if not identified and treated. The causative organism is Histoplasma capsulatum. There are three major types of the disease: 1) acute pulmonary histoplasmosis, 2) chronic pulmonary histoplasmosis, and 3) progressive disseminated histoplasmosis. A rare form of the disease is ocular histoplasmosis syndrome. While it can happen in anyone, it is more common among the immunosuppressed. The organism is found in soil, bird droppings, or bat guano.

The disease of Histoplasmosis may be asymptomatic but, if symptomatic, occurs 3-17 days following an exposure (about 14 days on average). Most patients have asymptomatic disease. People with disease symptoms will have a cough or flu-like symptoms. The chest x-ray will be normal about 40-70 percent of the time. Chronic histoplasmosis acts like tuberculosis and can affect multiple organs.

Figure 11 reveals the microscopy of histoplasmosis of the lungs:

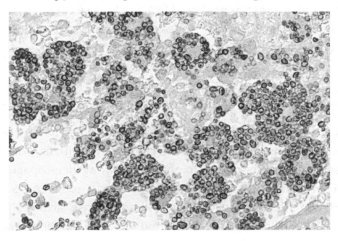

Figure 11

Symptoms of disseminated disease involves the mediastinum (mediastinitis), liver, spleen (hepatosplenomegaly), lymph nodes (lymphadenopathy), and the adrenal glands. Calcification occurs upon healing. Ocular histoplasmosis affects the eyes, causing scarring of the retina and choroid plexus. There will be loss of vision. Ocular disease usually happens in those who are immunocompromised.

Complications include respiratory failure, superior vena cava syndrome, pneumonia, fibrosing mediastinitis, and respiratory failure. There may be progressive lymph node fibrosis, obstruction of the pulmonary vessels, and retinal scarring. Smokers can develop a chronic form of the disease, called chronic cavitary histoplasmosis. Hard, calcified lymph nodes cause erosion of the airway walls, leading to hemoptysis.

The disease comes from inhaling the microconidia found in bird and bat droppings or soil but is not contagious from person to person. It forms a yeast at body temperatures and proliferates in the lungs. The microconidia get ingested inside the macrophages and live inside the phagosome. It transforms into a yeast and can grow inside the phagosome. The macrophages go to the lymph nodes and spread to different body organs. The fungus requires thiamine to proliferate. Eventually cell-mediated immunity develops and the macrophages contain the organism and eventually become calcified. Disseminated disease goes to bone, adrenal glands, spleen, liver, lungs, and mucocutaneous membranes.

Disseminated disease is generally chronic and may have oral lesions on the mucocutaneous membranes. The diagnosis can be made by looking for the fungus on a bronchoalveolar lavage, blood sample, or tissue biopsy of the affected tissues. It can also be found in urine or blood by looking for the antigen using PCR or ELISA. Antigens will cross-react with African histoplasmosis (caused by Histoplasma duboisii). It can also cross-react with blastomycosis and coccidioidomycosis. Skin testing can say if the person has been exposed but cannot identify the person with active disease (as this is an antibody test). A formal fungal culture is necessary to prove active disease. Serum antigen testing will be falsely negative before a month of developing disseminated disease. Urine antigen testing is a better diagnostic test.

Treatment is not necessary in immunocompetent people. The antifungal treatments for disease includes an initial trial of amphotericin B, followed by taking itraconazole orally. Liposomal amphotericin B is better than the antifungal made using deoxycholate. The major risk of taking amphotericin B is kidney failure. Treatment should last a year in serious cases but, in typical acute pulmonary histoplasmoses, treatment can last for 6-12 weeks. Less commonly used drugs for histoplasmosis include posaconazole, voriconazole, and fluconazole.

Cryptococcosis

Cryptococcosis or cryptococcal disease is a fungal disease that can be caused by either Cryptococcus gattii or Cryptococcus neoformans (although disease can be seen with C. grubii). It is caused by the inhalation of propagules in the environment. No one knows what the propagule actually is but it is believed to be a type of spore made by the organism. It is considered an AIDS defining disease and the second most common HIV-related disease in Africa. Patients at risk include HIV disease, lymphoma, cirrhosis, corticosteroid use, and sarcoidosis. It is found in the soil and inhaled.

There are three types of cryptococcosis, including cutaneous (wound-related) cryptococcosis, pulmonary cryptococcosis, and cryptococcal meningitis. Meningitis is believed to be a secondary disease from disseminated pulmonary cryptococcosis. While the disease can be seen in immunocompetent people, it is more likely to be seen in people who are immunocompromised (especially with problems with cell-mediated immunity). HIV disease is a common risk factor for disseminated disease. It is a highly fatal disease, even when treated. The mortality is 9 percent in developed countries but is 70 percent in sub-Saharan Africa, causing nearly a million deaths annually globally.

The diagnosis involves recognizing the clinical symptoms of tiredness, cough, fever, blurry vision, and headache. The symptoms develop gradually and can lead to meningitis or lung infections. The antigen can be detected in a tissue culture, CSF sample, sputum sample, or urine. Severe infections only can be detected with a positive blood culture. The CSF sample is stained with India ink. It has a 20 percent false-negative rate but can be cultured from the CSF. The most sensitive test for meningeal disease involves antigen testing of the CSF.

The treatment of cryptococcosis is IV amphotericin B and flucytosine (orally). People with AIDS have a high mortality rate of up to 70 percent after ten weeks but the same treatment is recommended. If flucytosine is unavailable, fluconazole can be used instead (with amphotericin B). Treatment will improve survival rates. Treatment starts with high doses of amphotericin B and oral flucytosine (or fluconazole). After one week, the oral treatment alone is used for a minimum of 8 weeks. AIDS patients should also be on antiretroviral therapy while being treated with the antifungal agents.

Coccidioidomycosis

Coccidioidomycosis can be called many names, including San Joaquin Valley fever, desert rheumatism, California fever, or Valley fever. The two main organisms involved are Coccidioides immitis and Coccidioides posadasii. It is an endemic disease in the Southwestern state, including Utah, Texas, New Mexico, Nevada, California, and Arizona, as well as in northern Mexico. It is found in the soil in desert-like areas and becomes a filamentous mold with spores during the rainy season. The spores (called arthroconidia) become airborne and, after inhalation, can cause disease. In endemic areas, it is a common cause of community-acquired pneumonia, especially after soil disruption. It is not contagious.

Only about 40 percent of patients will have symptoms, most often related to the lungs. The disease resembles pneumonia or bronchitis that lasts several weeks. It is responsible for 20 percent of community-acquired pneumonias in endemic areas. People feel feverish and fatigued, with symptoms of myalgias, arthralgias, rash, cough, and headaches. The fatigue can be long-lasting. It is called "desert rheumatism" because of its common presentation of erythema nodosum, fever, and arthralgias. About 3-5 percent of patients will develop chronic disease with disseminated infection (or just pneumonia). The meninges, joints, bones, and soft tissue can be involved in chronic cases. The most severe cases are associated with HIV disease.

The initial or acute phase is called Valley fever with the chronic phase being called disseminated coccidioidomycosis. The acute phase is often referred to as primary pulmonary coccidioidomycosis. Cutaneous disease is seen in disseminated coccidioidomycosis. Complications and death can occur in immunosuppressed people, who die from respiratory failure, lung nodules, disseminated disease, and bronchopleural fistulas. When disseminated, many body areas can be involved, including the skin, bladder, meninges, bones, joints, heart, and subcutaneous tissues.

Blastomycosis

This is often referred to as Gilchrist's disease or North American blastomycosis—an infection that can cause disease in humans, dogs, and cats. The organism is Blastomyces dermatitidis. It is endemic to many places in North America and is clinically similar to histoplasmosis. It can be seen in South America, India, Saudi Arabia, and Africa. It causes a flu-like disease with myalgias, arthralgias, fever, chills, headache, and dry cough that lasts for several days.

Blastomycosis can involve an acute pulmonary disease that resembles pneumonia. As a chronic disease, it resembles tuberculosis or lung cancer. Progressive and often fatal disease can cause adult respiratory distress syndrome and death in immunocompromised patients. Skin and bone lesions can result in clinical disease. Up to 40 percent of patients who are immunocompromised will have brain abscesses or meningitis, which can be fatal. It is found in moist soil and rotten wood.

Key Takeaways

- Most fungal diseases involve the inhalation of fungal spores that take root in the lungs.
- Fungal diseases can cause acute lung disease or result in disseminated disease, which is frequently fatal.
- There are antifungal medications that can be used to treat many fungal diseases but, when disseminated or severe, long-term treatment is required.
- Fungal diseases can be seen in immunocompetent and immunosuppressed patients but is more severe in immunocompromised patients.

Quiz

1. Where can most cases of systemic candidiasis be identified?
   a. Brain
   b. Heart
   c. Blood
   d. Bone

Answer: c. The most common place to find candidiasis in systemic disease is the blood.

2. What is the most common fungal infection in hospitalized patients?
   a. Systemic candidiasis
   b. Coccidiomycosis
   c. Histoplasmosis
   d. Cryptococcosis

Answer: a. Systemic candidiasis is the most common fungal infection in hospitalized patients.

3. What is the most common species of Candida isolated from human blood?
   a. C. glabrata
   b. C. parapsilosis
   c. C. tropicalis
   d. C. albicans

Answer: d. Candida albicans is the most common Candida species isolated from human blood.

4. What is the most common diagnostic tool in identifying an aspergillus infection?
   a. Antigen testing of blood
   b. Antibody testing of blood
   c. Fungal culture
   d. Tissue biopsy and silver staining

Answer: d. The best diagnostic tool is a tissue biopsy with silver staining, which will show the organism and its hyphae.

5. What is the mainstay of treatment in cases of allergic bronchopulmonary aspergillosis?
   a. Itraconazole
   b. Corticosteroids
   c. Amphotericin B
   d. Fluconazole

Answer: b. In cases of allergic bronchopulmonary aspergillosis, long-term corticosteroids are the major treatment of choice.

6. What fungal disease is also known as "Cave disease"?
   a. Histoplasmosis
   b. Disseminated Aspergillosis
   c. Coccidiomycosis

d. Cryptococcosis

Answer: a. Histoplasmosis has many names, including "Cave disease".

7. What area of the body does disseminated histoplasmosis not commonly affect?
    a. Kidneys
    b. Liver
    c. Spleen
    d. Adrenal glands

Answer: a. The disseminated forms of histoplasmosis travel to the bone, adrenal glands, spleen, liver, lungs, and mucocutaneous membranes. It doesn't settle in the kidneys.

8. Which test for histoplasmosis will not detect an active disease state?
    a. Tissue biopsy
    b. Urine antigen testing
    c. Skin testing
    d. Blood antigen testing

Answer: c. Skin testing is an antibody test that can detect antibodies for histoplasmosis but doesn't indicate if the person has active disease or not.

9. What is considered a common first-line agent for the treatment of acute pulmonary histoplasmosis?
    a. Posaconazole
    b. Voriconazole
    c. Fluconazole
    d. Amphotericin B

Answer: d. The treatment of choice as a first-line treatment for histoplasmosis is amphotericin B.

10. What is considered the most common reservoir for Coccidioides spores?
    a. Lake water
    b. Contaminated food
    c. Soil
    d. Lungs

Answer: c. The reservoir for Coccidioides is the soil. It is not contagious and is not necessarily caused by the ingestion of any kind of liquid or food.

Chapter 5: Common Protozoal Infections

Protozoa are unicellular, eukaryotic, and non-photosynthetic organisms. Only a few protozoa cause human disease, which are usually enteric in nature and cause the same symptoms from organism to organism. Other protozoal diseases, such as malaria, affect other body areas. Protozoal diseases are most common in developing countries of the world.

Malaria

Malaria is a common mosquito-borne disease affecting humans, primarily in tropical and equatorial areas of the world. The organism most commonly causing malaria is Plasmodium falciparum. Plasmodium falciparum is considered the main cause of malignant malaria; Plasmodium vivax is the most frequent cause of benign malaria; Plasmodium ovale is a less frequent cause of benign malaria; Plasmodium malariae is the cause of benign quartan malaria; and Plasmodium knowlesi is the cause of severe quotidian malaria in South East Asia.

The typical malaria symptoms (with an incubation period of 10-15 days) include fever, fatigue, headaches, and vomiting. The less common symptoms in severe disease include seizures, jaundice, coma, and death. Recurrences of the disease after several months is common. Individuals who have an initial infection will have milder infections later. If the individual isn't exposed to the protozoan again, they develop partial immunity to the organism.

Figure 12 depicts the life cycle of the malarial organism:

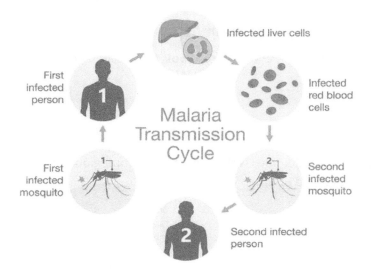

Figure 12

Malaria represents the most common mosquito-borne infection in the world. The female mosquito of the Anopheles species has the organism in its saliva and passes it onto people it bites. The organisms travel to the patient's liver and reproduce. The most common and deadly form is M. falciparum, with the other species causing milder disease. It is primarily diagnosed using a microscopic blood film analysis, although there are antigen-based diagnostic tests which expensive and not widely used.

The best way to prevent malaria is to use mosquito netting during sleep, mosquito repellents, and insecticides in the environment. Removing areas of standing water will decrease the disease incidence. Travelers to endemic are encouraged to take prophylactic medication, and a combination of sulfadoxine and pyrimethamine are used in babies and in women in the second or third trimesters of pregnancy (in endemic areas). Currently there is no effective vaccine for the disease.

The disease is endemic to several tropical and subtropical areas, including Asia, Latin America, and Sub-Saharan Africa. The prevalence of malaria is about 300 million people with about 700,000 deaths from the disease. Ninety percent of cases and deaths happen in Africa, being more prevalent in poorer parts of the world. It has a big economic effect on African economy, causing $12 billion USD per year to be spent on the disease.

The symptoms can still occur in people who've taken preventative measures but will happen later than the typical 10-15-day incubation period. All malaria cases are similar to flu-like illnesses but more severe cases can develop other symptoms, similar to sepsis or gastroenteritis. Very severe cases will have hemoglobinuria, jaundice, hemolytic anemia, flu-like symptoms, retinal disease, and seizures.

There are three classic paroxysmal symptoms seen differently in different strains of the disease. Both P. vivax and P. ovale cause coldness alternating with sweating and fever every two days (called tertian fever), while P. malariae causes fever alternating with coldness every three days (called quartan fever). P. falciparum causes alternating symptoms every 36-48 hours or a continuous fever. Almost all severe cases are caused by P. falciparum. When cerebral malaria occurs, it can lead to a number of neurological symptoms, including seizures and coma.

Severe complications of malaria include respiratory distress (occurring in 25-40 percent of cases) and severe anemia. Pregnant women and children have more severe disease, and patients with HIV disease have an increased risk of death. If there is hemoglobinuria, this can be called Blackwater fever, resulting in renal failure. Hepatomegaly and splenomegaly can occur in severe disease, and some patients can develop a severe bleeding disorder, hemorrhaging, and shock. Affected pregnant women are at risk of miscarriages and stillbirths.

About 75 percent of cases are secondary to Plasmodium falciparum, with P. vivax causing about 20 percent of infections. The rest of cases ae caused by either P. malariae, P. knowlesi, or P. vivax. Most of the deaths are secondary to P. falciparum, although some can be caused by P. vivax. The incidence of P. vivax cases is higher outside of Africa.

The treatment of malaria involves multiple drug regimens (because of resistances). The primary treatment is a type of artemisinin combined with lumefantrine, mefloquine, or sulfadoxine/pyrimethamine. If an artemisinin is not available, a combination of doxycycline and quinine can be used. There are known resistances to chloroquine and artemisinin. The combination treatments are effective 90 percent of the time. Quinine and clindamycin can be used in early pregnancy with artemisinin-based therapies used in the latter parts of the pregnancy. Patients with a P. vivax infection require dual treatment of the blood infection and for clearance of the organism from the liver. The use of tafenoquine is recommended to prevent relapsing disease in P. vivax infections. Severe P. falciparum malaria causes death in 10-50 percent of cases, especially with cerebral disease. In such cases, IV antimalarial drugs are recommended.

Toxoplasmosis

Toxoplasmosis is a protozoal disease caused by Toxoplasma gondii. It generally causes no symptoms but a few patients can have several weeks of a flu-like illness (with myalgias and lymphadenitis). Immunosuppressed patients can have neurological symptoms, such as seizures, and pregnant mothers are at risk of congenital toxoplasmosis affecting their unborn child.

There are a couple of ways to get the disease. The most common way is to eat improperly cooked food containing the cysts of the protozoan. The other common ways to get the disease include exposure in utero and exposure to cat feces in litter boxes. It is rarely transmitted via a blood transfusion but cannot otherwise be spread from person to person.

Figure 13 indicates what the toxoplasma organism looks like microscopically:

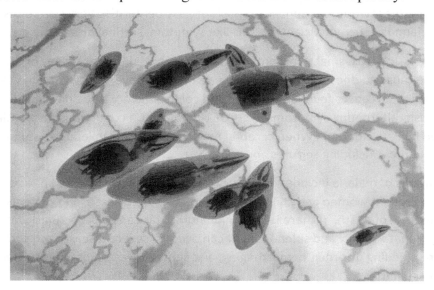

Figure 13

On average about 50 percent of people in the world will have antibodies against toxoplasma but will have had no symptoms. In the US, about 23 percent of people are affected and, in other areas of the world, about 95 percent of the population have positive antibodies. About 200,000 cases of congenital disease occur in the world per year.

There are different stages to the infection with toxoplasmosis. In acute disease, most people have no symptoms or just flu-like symptoms lasting about a month. Immunosuppressed patients can have pulmonary involvement and neurological symptoms (including seizures and confusion). Ocular toxoplasmosis can be seen in immunocompromised people, causing necrotizing retinochoroiditis. Encephalitis or ocular toxoplasmosis can be seen in newborns with congenital disease. The classic symptoms seen in babies with congenital toxoplasmosis include chorioretinitis, hydrocephalus, and intracranial artherosclerosis.

Latent toxoplasmosis involves having tissue cysts called bradyzoites in the body, which can form lesions in the heart, CNS, skeletal muscles, or lungs. The cysts in the brain do not go away so that infants infected in utero can have CNS problems later in life. Subtle CNS problems have been reported in immunocompetent hosts.

The third phase is cutaneous toxoplasmosis, which involves itchy skin lesions, more common in newborns. It can be diagnosed by doing a biopsy of the lesions showing the tachyzoite from of Toxoplasma gondii in the skin.

The diagnosis of toxoplasmosis can be made in several ways. It can be hard to tell the difference between the infection and primary CNS lymphoma and other infectious diseases. The organism can be detected in the blood, CSF, or amniotic fluid by a polymerase chain reaction test. This will not detect cysts in latent disease. Serology for the IgG antibodies to toxoplasma can be done to see if the patient has had the disease. They can be detected within a week of infection onset and last for life (so it doesn't detect active disease necessarily).

IgM antibody testing can detect active disease within a week of symptom onset but can still be seen months or years after an active infection so it isn't that effective in detecting acute disease. Besides PCR testing of amniotic fluid, a neonatal exam and cord blood evaluation can detect disease.

Treatment is only recommended for patients with immunosuppression. Acute cases can be treated with sulfadiazine, pyrimethamine, clindamycin, or spiramycin (especially in early pregnancy). A combination of pyrimethamine/sulfadiazine and leucovorin are used in the latter parts of pregnancy for active disease. These drugs are ineffective in ridding the body of the bradyzoites seen in latent disease. A combination of clindamycin and atovaquone is used for latent disease.

Women with acute toxoplasmosis have a 30 percent chance of passing the disease onto their fetus. The transmission rate increases with increased gestational age. Spiramycin can prevent transmission of the protozoan in the first trimester. After this, a combination of pyrimethamine/sulfadiazine and folinic acid can be used until delivery. Early fetal transmission is associated with the worst outcomes for the infant.

Leishmaniasis

Leishmaniasis is a protozoal disease caused by Leishmania. Cutaneous leishmaniasis in Asia and Europe are caused by the species L. major, L. tropica, and L. aethiopica. In other parts of the world, the most common species in cutaneous disease is L. mexicana.

Mucocutaneous disease is caused by L. braziliensis. Visceral leishmaniasis is caused by the L. donovani complex (L. donovani, L. infantum syn. L. chagasi). The cutaneous disease involves just skin ulcers; the mucocutaneous disease involves ulcerations around and in the mouth and nose; the visceral disease has skin ulcers followed by systemic disease (anemia, fever, hepatomegaly, and splenomegaly).

Figure 14 describes the appearance of the Leishmania organism:

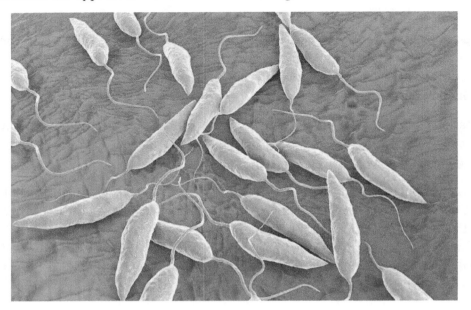

Figure 14

As it is mainly transmitted by the bite of a sand fly, the best prevention is spraying sleeping nets with insecticides and treating patients as early in the disease as possible to prevent person-to-person transmission. It occurs in poorer parts of the world and mainly tropical areas. About 4-12 million people have the disease at any given point in time. About 2 million new patients are identified each year with up to 50 thousand deaths per year. Most cases are in Africa, Asia, South America, Central America, and Southern Europe.

The main symptom is skin sores that take weeks to months to develop after being bitten. The cutaneous disease is the most common type. It heals within a couple of years, leaving a scar. Diffuse disease is possible and looks like leprosy. Mucocutaneous disease has the addition of mucosal ulcers of the nose and mouth. Visceral disease is called black fever, which can be fatal. Chronic visceral disease is possible, occurring months to years after the infection.

The disease diagnosis involves visualization of Leishman-Donovan bodies (amastigotes) from the blood, bone marrow, lymph nodes, skin lesions, or spleen aspirates. There is a special Leishman stain that can detect the disease in monocytes of the spleen or blood or in tissue macrophages. Some amastigotes can be detected freely in the tissues. There are ELISA tests, direct agglutination tests, and antigen tests that will detect the disease but they are rarely done because they are not very sensitive or specific for the disease. The PCR test is sensitive and specific, having the advantage of not being as painful as a tissue aspirate. It is possible to be spread from human to human.

The treatment of leishmaniasis depends on the geographic location, type of infection, and species involved. Liposomal amphotericin B is used for visceral disease in some parts of the world with a single dose effective in 95 percent of cases. Leishmaniasis is difficult to cure in Africa and India because of resistances but miltefosine can treat both visceral and cutaneous leishmaniasis in certain cases.

African sleeping sickness

This is called African trypanosomiasis or sleeping sickness; it is an insect-borne protozoal disease caused by Trypanosoma brucei (of which there are two strains: T. b. rhodesiense and T. b. gambiense). Both types stem from the bite of a tsetse fly in rural parts of Africa. There are two stages to the disease. The first stage involves headaches, pruritis, fever, and arthralgias. The incubation period is 1-3 weeks. This stage is seen with massive enlargement of the lymph nodes (called the Winterbottom's sign) and a chancre at the site of the bite. Untreated first-stage disease leads to kidney failure, heart failure, anemia, and endocrine disease.

The second stage or "neurological stage" happens weeks or months later and involves incoordination, neuropathy, confusion, and abnormalities of the sleep-wake cycle. It can be diagnosed by looking for the parasite in the blood or lymph fluid. The organism can be detected in the CSF of patients with second-stage disease. The second-stage of the disease has a 100 percent mortality rate without treatment. The disease will involve progressive mental deterioration, coma, multisystem organ failure, and death. Even with treatment, any neurological changes found will be permanent and untreatable.

Prevention of second stage (severe) disease involves screening people with possible first stage disease and treating positive patients as the disease is easier to treat in the early stages. The medications pentamidine and suramin are used to treat the disease in the first stage, while eflornithine or a combination of eflornithine and nifurtimox are used in second stage disease. Treatment averts certain death in second stage disease.

The disease is primarily seen in sub-Saharan Africa. The prevalence is about 11,000 people with about 3400 deaths per year (because of treatment). It seems to occur in outbreaks, primarily in the Republic of Congo and Uganda. It is carried in cows as well as humans.

The most accurate test for African sleeping sickness is identifying trypanosomes in the blood, bone marrow, lymph node aspirates, or chancre. It will only be seen in the CSF with second-stage disease. Antibody testing is available but is inaccurate for diagnostic purposes. A wet prep can be used to detect motile organisms, while a fixed prep can be stained and examined for dead organisms in the fluid or tissues. Concentrates of blood and body fluid are necessary to see the organism.

The treatment needs to be fairly aggressive for both stages. IV or IM pentamidine is used for first-stage T. b. gambiense and IV suramin is used for first-stage T. b. rhodesiense. Second-stage T. b. gambiense requires IV eflornithine and nifurtimox. Second-line treatment is with IV melarsoprol, which has a risk of death for the drug alone.

Chagas disease

This is also referred to as American trypanosomiasis. It is a tropical protozoal disease caused by Trypanosoma cruzi. It is spread by Triatominae or "kissing bugs". Triatominae are called kissing bugs because they tend to bite people on the face and defecate on the person after biting them. It is the feces that cause the infection. Some patients will have localized eye swelling from an infection near the eye.

Figure 15 describes the life cycle of Chagas disease:

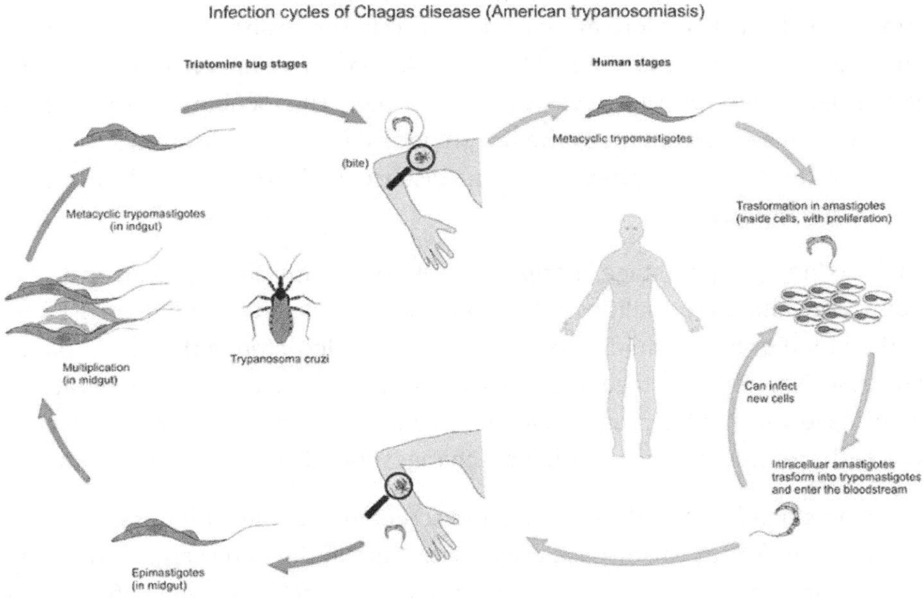

Infection cycles of Chagas disease (American trypanosomiasis)

Figure 15

The course of the disease varies over time with early stage disease being mild or absent (with swollen lymph nodes, headaches, fever, and swelling at the insect bite site). Rare cases of acute disease will cause myocarditis or meningoencephalitis, leading to death, especially in patients who are immunosuppressed. While symptoms resolve in weeks, the organism is still present and survive within the human host, causing an indeterminant length of chronic disease.

After about 2-3 months, the disease become chronic, which is also asymptomatic in 60-70 percent of cases. The rest of patients have symptoms that don't develop for 10-30 years. When they do develop symptoms (called determinate chronic Chagas disease), it involves things like heart failure (from dilated cardiomyopathy), enlargement of the colon (megacolon), or enlargement of the esophagus (megaesophagus). The symptoms in the late stage can be fatal. About 10 percent of patients do not have an asymptomatic indeterminate phase but go on to symptomatic late stage Chagas disease. Untreated late stage disease is often fatal.

While most cases of Chagas disease are spread by kissing bugs, it can be spread via blood transfusion, eating food with the protozoa in it, organ transplant, or in utero. Like many cases, it can be seen in the blood samples of patients with early disease and with antibody testing in late or chronic disease. It can cause stillbirths and significant cause of such in places like Brazil.

The only way to diagnose Chagas disease with any certainty is to do a direct microscopic evaluation of fresh anticoagulated blood for motile protozoa or by staining blood smears with a Giemsa dye. There is a xenodiagnosis that can be done in which the bugs are fed patient's blood and then examined for their GI content of T. cruzi. It can also be inoculated into mice and cultured with a special media for protozoal species. There are immunoassays for the parasite that can differentiate between strains of the pathogen. There are indirect fluorescence tests, ELISA tests, PCR tests, and radio-immunoassays, of which the direct visualization or xenodiagnoses are the most accurate methods of detection.

There is no vaccine for the disease but it can be treated early with benznidazole or nifurtimox with cure happening in early cases. Medications for chronic cases may prevent end-stage disease but they will not cure the disease. Side effects of the drugs limit their use as they can cause GI irritation, skin rashes, and neurological toxicity.

Both drugs used for the treatment of T. cruzi are limited in their ability to completely get rid of the parasite from the body, partly because of drug resistance and partly because it is very difficult to get rid of the protozoa from chronically-infected patients. About 90 percent of infants can be cured and about 60-85 percent of adults can be cured with acute disease. The longer an adult has the chronic form of the disease, the more difficult it is to cure. However, treatment can delay the onset of complications.

The total number of people in the world who have had the disease is about 6.6 million, with an annual death rate of about 8000 per year, with many not recognizing they have the disease. It is mainly found in tropical areas but in rare cases, has been seen in other parts of the world.

Complications of the disease include arrhythmias, which require pacemakers and medications to control heart failure. Surgery is necessary for megacolon. Heart transplantation surgery is a common treatment for severe cases. There is no evidence that taking immunosuppressive therapy will worsen the disease after the transplant.

Giardiasis

Giardiasis is also called "beaver fever" and is a protozoal disease caused by Giardia lamblia. It is asymptomatic in only 10 percent of cases. The rest will get symptoms of abdominal pain, diarrhea, and weight loss. Less common symptoms include nausea, vomiting, fever, and hematochezia. The incubation period is 1-3 weeks, while the infection time without treatment is about six weeks. The symptoms can develop in as little as one day after exposure but averages 9-15 days. The part of the body affected is mainly the duodenum and jejunum, interfering with the absorption of nutrients. Milk cannot be digested and carbohydrates are poorly absorbed. Vitamin B12 is also poorly absorbed.

The disease is passed via the fecal oral route so that cysts from the organism in feces contaminate food or water the person consumes. Travel in the developing part of the world, changing an infected person's diaper, or eating food without cooking it properly will increase the risk. Having a dog increases the risk. Cysts can survive cold weather for a maximum of three months. Giardiasis tends to happen more frequently in the summer months when people are outdoors more and engaging in wilderness activities.

Figure 16 shows the microscopic appearance of the Giardia organism:

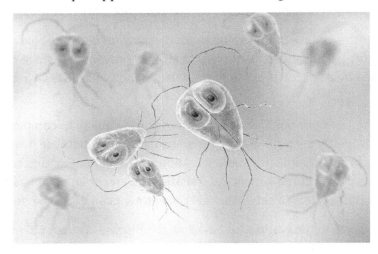

Figure 16

The diagnosis of giardiasis involves antigen testing of stool specimens. This involves the most sensitive way to test for the disorder. Another stool test is a trichrome stain of the stool as well as visual examination of the stool for motile trophozoites or for the presence of cysts. There is a test involving swallowing a capsule attached to the mouth with a string. The capsule enters the small bowel and is withdrawn, bringing up trophozoites for examination under the microscope.

There is actually no need to treat the disease as it will resolve on its own. Metronidazole is the first-line treatment for symptomatic disease; however, tinidazole and nitazoxanide are the only two drugs actually approved by the FDA for giardiasis. The advantage of using tinidazole is only a single dose is required. There are known resistances to all of the drugs for giardiasis so other drugs may be necessary to manage resistant disease. Paromomycin is the drug of choice for pregnancy as it is not absorbed by the GI tract very well. Metronidazole can be used after the first trimester of pregnancy as well.

The best prevention is good hygiene, and the best treatment is either metronidazole or tinidazole. Lactose intolerance develops during an infection so milk should be avoided. This is the most common protozoal disease in the world, affecting about 280 million people per year across the globe. As many as 30 percent of people have the disease in developing countries, while 7 percent of people get the disease in the developed world.

Key Takeaways

- Protozoal infections can be in the bloodstream or the GI tract, leading to a wide variety of symptoms.
- Some protozoal infections are uniformly fatal unless they are treated with medications.
- The majority of protozoal diseases are passed through an insect vector; however, others can be developed after ingesting the cysts.
- Giardiasis is the most common protozoal infection in the world, followed by malaria.

Quiz

1. Which species is considered the main cause of malaria?
   a. Plasmodium vivax
   b. Plasmodium falciparum
   c. Plasmodium ovale
   d. Plasmodium malariae

Answer: b. The major cause of malaria is Plasmodium falciparum; however, the other choices do cause the disease in less common situations.

2. What is the most common way to diagnose malaria?
   a. Antigen testing of serum
   b. Antibody testing of serum
   c. Blood culture for Plasmodium
   d. Peripheral blood smear evaluation

Answer: d. A peripheral blood smear evaluation will show the organisms in the bloodstream and is the most efficient and cheapest way to detect disease.

3. What is the average incubation period of Plasmodium falciparum?
   a. 2-4 days
   b. 7-10 days
   c. 10-15 days
   d. 15-40 days

Answer: c. The incubation period of Plasmodium falciparum before symptoms of malaria develop is about 10-15 days.

4. What is the best way to detect congenital toxoplasmosis in a fetus?
   a. PCR testing of the amniotic fluid
   b. IgM antibody testing of the mother's serum
   c. IgG antibody testing of the mother's serum
   d. PCR testing of the mother's blood

Answer: a. PCR testing of the amniotic fluid will be fairly sensitive in detecting congenital toxoplasmosis. Testing the mother will not necessarily be effective to determine if the infection has been passed to the fetus.

5. What organism is most likely to cause mucocutaneous leishmaniasis?
   a. L. donovani
   b. L. infantum
   c. L. chagasi
   d. L. braziliensis

Answer: d. The only organism that will lead to mucocutaneous leishmaniasis is Leishmania braziliensis. The others will cause visceral leishmaniasis.

6. What is the most common classification of leishmaniasis?
   a. Mucocutaneous disease
   b. Cutaneous disease
   c. Visceral disease
   d. Cerebral disease

Answer: b. The most common classification of leishmaniasis is cutaneous disease, which causes skin eruptions that may be focal or systemic.

7. What is the estimated mortality rate in untreated second-stage African sleeping sickness?
   a. 10 percent
   b. 25 percent
   c. 60 percent
   d. 100 percent

Answer: d. Untreated second-stage African sleeping sickness is 100 percent fatal if not treated aggressively with anti-protozoal medications.

8. Where can trypanosomes be seen in second-stage African sleeping sickness that cannot be seen in the first stage of the disease?
   a. Lymph nodes
   b. Cerebrospinal fluid
   c. Chancre
   d. Spleen

Answer: b. The finding of trypanosomes in the CSF is 100 percent indicative of second-stage disease versus first-stage disease.

9. What finding is not seen in late stage Chagas disease?
   a. Cardiac enlargement
   b. Esophageal enlargement
   c. ARDS
   d. Colon enlargement

Answer: c. Late-stage Chagas disease involves enlargement of the heart, esophagus, and colon.

10. What disease represents the most common protozoal disease in the world?
    a. African sleeping sickness
    b. Chagas disease
    c. Malaria
    d. Giardiasis

Answer: d. Giardiasis is the most common protozoal disease in the world, affecting about 280 million individuals.

Chapter 6: Common Parasitic Infections

This chapter will discuss common parasitic diseases, including those caused by endoparasites (which cause internal disease) and those caused by ectoparasites (which cause external human disease). Parasites cause a type of human disease called a parasitosis. Although most parasites do not cause diseases, there are some parasites that can infect almost all living organisms.

Cestodiasis

Cestodiasis is the medical term for a tapeworm infection of the GI tract caused by a flatworm or cestode. The larvae are grouped in cysts found in undercooked meat, which accounts for most tapeworm infestations. After the larvae are ingested, they can hatch and grow into an extremely large tapeworm.

Figure 17 shows what a tapeworm looks like:

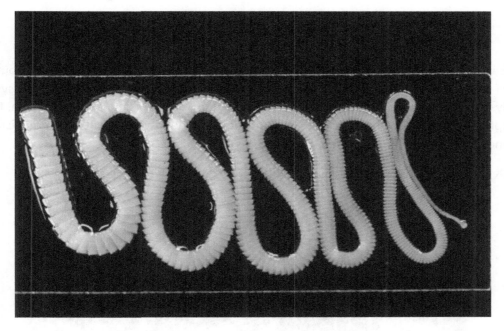

Figure 17

Most people have no associated symptoms with a tapeworm infestation, except for the occasional anorexia, diarrhea, and upper abdominal pain. However, the fish tapeworm may also cause anemia. A tapeworm infection may first me notices by the patient after the passage of worm segments in the stool (which are often moving). Rare symptoms include intestinal obstruction or neurological symptoms from T. solium, which is associated with larvae in the brain causing neurocysticercosis. Nervous-system related tapeworm infestations can last for several years before symptoms develop.

Each tapeworm egg has the potential to cause an infection. Segments are called proglottids and contain thousands of tapeworm eggs. The eggs become larvae after being ingested and travel to the lungs or liver, forming cysts. This is especially seen with cysticercosis (the pork tapeworm) or echinococcosis (dog or sheep tapeworms).

Raw or undercooked meat from a number of sources can lead to cestodiasis. The larvae are grouped into cysts called coenuri in the muscle tissue. The larvae can grow in the intestinal tract up to a size of 55 feet long and a survival rate of up to 25 years. They can attach to the inside of the GI tract or can pass through the GI tract unaffected (living out the entire life cycle in the same person). Many tapeworms is can also be passed from one person to another. Reinfection can occur even when being treated for the infestation (more common if the person has poor hygiene).

The pork tapeworm is called T. solium; the beef tapeworm is called T. saginata; the fish tapeworm is called Diphyllobothrium; the dwarf tapeworm is called Hymenolepsis. The sheep and cow genus (causing disease in these animals) is called Echinococcus. All except for the fish tapeworm have four suckers on the head (scolex) that attaches to the inner GI lining.

Often, only a single dose of medication is required to successfully deworm and infected patient. The drug of choice for tapeworm infestations is praziquantel, although Niclosamide can also be used.

Ascariasis

Ascariasis is a roundworm infection caused by the parasitic worm Ascaris lumbricoides. About 85 percent of patients will be asymptomatic, especially when the infestation is mild. Common symptoms include dyspnea and fever, followed by abdominal distention, diarrhea, and abdominal pain. In children, later symptoms include learning difficulties, malnutrition, and poor weight gain. The organisms secrete antienzymes that overwhelm the host's digestive enzymes.

Figure 18 shows roundworms microscopically:

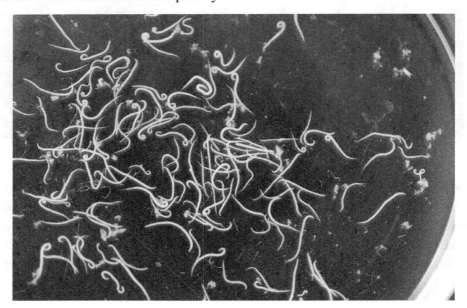

Figure 18

The infection develops via the fecal oral route so poor hygiene plays a role. The eggs are ingested and go deep into the abdominal wall. The larvae travel to the lungs and pass up the trachea, where they are coughed up and re-swallowed. At the second pass in the GI tract, they become adult roundworms. Roundworms can be transmitted from soil with the eggs, thus good handwashing with soap and water are good preventative measures. Treating everyone at regular intervals in high risk patients (with 20 percent or more of the people infected) is recommended.

Most people are infected with a small number of ascaris roundworms with just a few people heavily infested. This means that many are asymptomatic. There may be damage to the viscera, peritonitis, and visceral inflammation, splenomegaly or hepatomegaly. The lungs may become inflamed. Loeffler's syndrome involves lung inflammation, associated with pulmonary infiltrates and eosinophilia. Large numbers of worms can ball together, causing an intestinal blockage and bowel obstruction. They can obstruct the pancreatic ducts, leading to acute pancreatitis. Cholecystitis and cholangitis may also occur.

Roundworm infections may exacerbate or cause dust mites and shrimp allergies, secondary to a shared antigen. Other associated symptoms may include anorexia and malabsorption secondary to the lack of brush border enzymes and villi flattening. The only way to identify the disease is test for worms or eggs in a stool sample. The patient themselves may also see the worm in their stool. Larvae may be detected on a sputum sample in the pulmonary phase of the disease. Eosinophilia may be present, but isn't specific.

There is no vaccine for the disease and is possible to be reinfected. Common medications used to treat roundworms are ascaricides including mebendazole, albendazole, pyrantel pamoate, and levamisole. The main risk of pyrantel pamoate is that it can cause intestinal obstruction. Albendazole cannot be used in pregnancy or in babies. Thiabendazole can cause the roundworm to migrate up the esophagus so it is often combined with piperazine. Second-line agents include tribendimidine and nitazoxanide. Surgery is used to treat a bowel obstruction.

Around a billion people are infected, especially in sub-Saharan Africa, Asia, and Latin America. It causes about 2700 deaths per year. Prevention includes improved hygiene and not using human feces as a form of fertilizer. Mass drug administration of a single dose of mebendazole or albendazole can be given to all children in high risk communities to decrease the incidence of the disease.

Filariasis

Filariasis is another parasitic illness caused by specific roundworms of the Filarioidea classification. These can be spread by mosquito bites and black flies. There are eight known filarial round worms that use the human host. They represent three major types.

The first type is called lymphatic filariasis, caused by one of three worms: Brugia timori, Brugia malayi, or Wuchereria bancrofti. They live in the lymph system (lymph nodes primarily). They can lead to elephantiasis. The most common symptom in lymphatic disease is elephantiasis secondary to obstruction of the lymph system. It mainly affects the lower extremities. Different types of filariasis cause elephantiasis in different places. For example, Wuchereria bancrofti causes breast, vulva, arm, and leg elephantiasis, while Brugia timori does not affect the genitalia.

Figure 19 shows an individual with elephantiasis from filariasis:

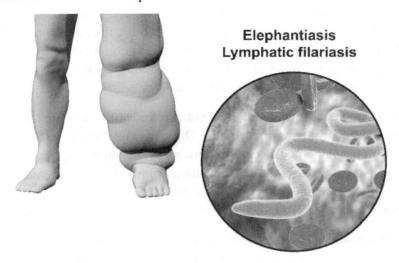

Figure 19

The second type is subcutaneous filariasis, caused by the loa loa (eye worm), Mansonella streptocerca, or Oncherocera volvulus. These live in the skin (in the subcutaneous tissue). The disease from L. loa is called loa loa filariasis, while O. volvulus is the cause of "river blindness". These patients will have urticaria, arthritis, and papules, as well as hypopigmented or hyperpigmented macules on the skin. River blindness is one of the leading causes of blindness throughout the globe.

Serous cavity filariasis can be caused by Mansonella perstans and Mansonella ozzardi. They live in the serous cavity of the abdomen. The symptoms of this type of infestation is similar to subcutaneous disease except for the addition of abdominal pain.

The larvae can be found in the host's blood stream, where they are picked up by the insect vector. The adult worms usually reside in a specific tissue. The patients with microfilaremic disease have obvious microfilariae in the bloodstream, while amicrofilaremic disease involves no obvious microfilariae in the bloodstream. Performing antigen testing on may be helpful in confirming the diagnosis of amicrofilaremic disease.

The main diagnosis is finding the larvae on blood smears stained with Giemsa, which is the gold standard of testing. A finger prick is all that's required to identify the disease state. The time of the blood draw depends on the timing of the life cycle of the organism. It doesn't work for M. streptocerca or O. volvulus, are only found in the skin, thus skin biopsies may show evidence of the disease.

Other methods that aren't a gold standard include PCR testing and antigenic testing of the blood, which are mainly effective in cases of amicrofilaremic situations. It can be drawn at any time of the day and will be relatively sensitive. A lymph node aspirate can be done to show the presence of microfilariae in the lymphatic cases of the disease. An x-ray of chronic cases will show calcification of adult worms in the lymph tissue.

The treatment outside of the US is albendazole and ivermectin (combined). These are strictly microfilaricides and won't treat the adult worms. Doxycycline can help patients with elephantiasis by destroying the symbiotic bacteria that live inside the adult worms. It destroys the ability of the worm to reproduce.

Scabies

Scabies is called the "seven-year itch" and is an ectoparasite that causes a contagious skin infection. The organism is the mite Sarcoptes scabiei and the main symptoms are extreme itchiness and a papular rash. The incubation period between infestation and symptoms is 2-6 weeks. A secondary infection takes only 24 hours to become symptomatic. It can be a total-body rash or a rash of specific body areas. Itching is worse at night and leads to secondary bacterial infections.

Figure 20 shows a scabies infection of the upper extremity:

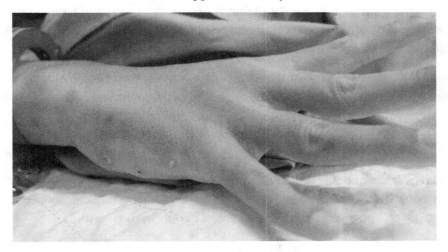

Figure 20

Along with ringworm and impetigo, scabies is one of the top three skin disorders of children. About 200 people have scabies per year, which effects people of all ages. It is seen more often in tropical climates and in the developing world.

The mites will burrow into the skin, and deposit their eggs. The symptoms of scabies are actually secondary to an allergic reaction to the mites. Only 10-15 mites cause an active infestation. It is passed from person to person though prolonged contact. It can spread without the patient having symptoms. It is seen more often in crowded conditions. Crusted scabies is more severe and occurs in the immunosuppressed person. Millions of mites are involved, making the person much more contagious. The mite is too small to see with the naked eye so the diagnosis is clinical.

The actual symptoms stem mostly stem from the cell-mediated response to the allergic component of the mite. IgE antibodies are present in the bloodstream and at the infection site. Because of prior exposure, the allergic response is much faster the second and subsequent times of reinfection.

Patients with HIV disease, people on immunosuppressants, and people with cancer can develop crusted scabies. It used to be known as Norwegian scabies. There are many more mites that overwhelm the body's immune system, spreading everywhere but the face. These aren't any more virulent, just more prevalent. Patients have milder itching, scaly rashes, and thick crusts of skin containing huge numbers of mites. It is difficult to treat because topical application of commonly used anti-scabies medicines can't get to the mites.

A variety of medications can treat scabies, including topical permethrin, crotamiton, and lindane. Oral ivermectin will also work. Sexual contacts and household contacts should be treated simultaneously. Bedding and clothing will need to be washed (in hot water) and dried on high heat. Mites only survives for three days outside the body so clothing and bedding used before this time doesn't need washing. The allergy-mediated symptoms last about 2-4 weeks after treatment. Retreatment may be necessary if symptoms persist beyond this time.

The most effective treatment for scabies is permethrin—the first-line agent for the infestation. It is applied from the neck down before bedtime and washed off 8-14 hours later. The entire body surface must be covered. One treatment is usually all that is necessary as eggs and hatchlings are killed along with the adult mite. Some physicians recommend retreatment 3-7 days later to make sure everything was killed. Multiple treatments are necessary to treat the crusted form of the disease.

Oral ivermectin involves a single dose of the medication. It is used on people older than six years of age. Topical ivermectin preps are available but they are not yet FDA-approved for human use.

Pediculosis Pubis

This is also known as crabs or pubic lice. It is caused by Pthirus pubis, a type of parasitic insect that primarily affects pubic hair. It can also live on the eyelashes (causing pediculosis ciliaris). It is intensely itchy in the pubic region and affects about 2 percent of people in the world.

Figure 21 shows the pubic lice organism on a hair:

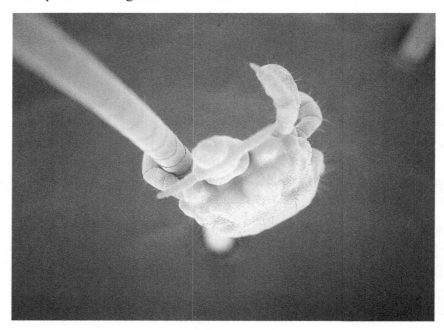

Figure 21

The itching actually comes from a hypersensitivity reaction to the saliva of the organism, which leads to more intense symptoms about two weeks after the first infestation. Nits or live lice can be seen without a microscope with adult lice seen crawling in the pubic area.

The disease is commonly spread through sexual activity and not commonly found in children. It can only survive for a short time away from the humidity and warmth of the skin. There are three life stages of the louse: the egg or nit, the nymph stage, and the adult organism. Nits are attached to the hair shaft and take 6-10 days to hatch. The nymph is an immature louse that grows to maturity in 2-3 weeks. They feed on blood. Adults have six legs of which the two front legs are pinchers. It will die in 1-2 days if not attached to human skin. About 30 eggs are laid during the 3-4 weeks that the adult survives. There is no other host except for humans. Clothing and bedding play a minor role in passing on the disease.

The diagnosis of the disease is purely clinical as nits, nymphs, or adult lice can be visualized with or without a microscope. Patients should have other STD evaluations if they have crabs. The treatment involves topical agents, such as permethrin, or a combination of pyrethrin and piperonyl butoxide. These are available over the counter. The topical cream or lotion is left on the skin for an hour before removing. A second treatment should take place in a weeks' time to kill newly hatched nymphs as eggs don't get killed with the medication. Lindane is a second-line therapy because it can be toxic. It shouldn't be used on people with dermatitis as this may cause too much of the medication to enter the bloodstream. It shouldn't be used in kids, the elderly, or people with seizures that aren't well controlled. Bedding and clothing should be washed and dried with high heat. Sexual partners should be treated as well.

Pediculosis Capitus

A pediculosis capitus infection is also referred to as head lice. It is an infection of the hair on the head with the head louse called "Pediculosis humanus capitus". Itching from lice bites is the main symptom of the disease. Itching may not develop until six weeks after the infestation. Reinfestation causes more rapid symptoms. Head lice may spread other diseases in Africa but this is not common in Europe or North America.

Figure 22 shows nits seen with head lice:

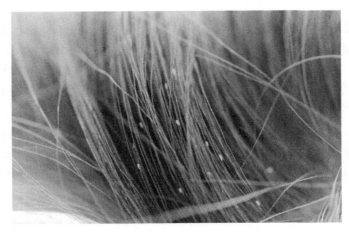

Figure 22

The disease is extremely common, affecting about 1-20 percent of children throughout the world. About 6-12 million kids get the disease in the US each year. Girls are more likely to be infected when compared to boys. It doesn't cause serious disease but will be extremely itchy. Rare symptoms include fever and lymphadenopathy. Bacterial infections from itching is possible.

The spread of the disease is by direct contact with an infected person's hair, combs, or things like hats and scarves. It isn't strongly related to hygiene. They can survive for three days outside of the contact of human skin. It can be diagnosed by seeing live lice. Seeing empty nits are not enough to make the diagnosis. The areas most likely to show the organism are the nape of the neck and the area behind the ears. Again, live lice indicate an active infection and not the nits.

Treatments include combing the hair with a fine-tooth come to remove the nits or shaving the head which also eliminates the nits. Topical treatments include ivermectin, malathion, and dimethicone. Dimethicone is a type of silicone oil that is a preferred treatment due to the limited side effects. Permethrin has been used historically but there is a lot of insect resistance to the drug.

The goal of treatment and prevention involves the regular evaluation of he child's head for live lice. The treatment is easier in the early stages of the disease with topical agents. High risk patients are kids between 4 and 15 years old. Infected clothing, combs, hairbrushes, bedding, and towels should be left outside for two days and not used, or washed at 60 degrees for thirty minutes and dried on high. There is no need to treat potentially infected furniture or mattresses.

Pediculosis Corporis

Pediculosis corporis is also known as body lice, pediculosis vestimenti, and vagabond's disease. It is a skin condition caused by Pediculosis corporis (body louse) that lays its eggs in the seams of clothing. Typical signs and symptoms include intense itching. Body lice can transmit other diseases, such as epidemic typhus, relapsing fever, and trench fever.

Major risk factors for the disease include contact with an infected person, bedding, clothing, or towels. It is not a common disease, seen mainly in homeless people who don't bathe often or change clothing often. Secondary transmission of the different bloodborne diseases are less likely to occur unless there is a prison situation, war, or natural disaster.

The management of body lice is to improve hygiene, including washing clothes and bathing once a week or more. Everything infected should be washed in hot water and dried on high heat. If hygiene can be maintained, the organism will die off without treatment but it needs treatment if this can't be done. Topical pediculocide treatment is recommended. Not wearing infected clothing for a week will also protect the person and delouse the clothing.

Pediculocide treatment involves powder dusting with DDT, malathion, or permethrin. Topical ivermectin used on days 0, 7, and 14 (three doses total) will help but won't eradiate the disease. The problem does not need anything special if the clothing and body are washed more frequently.

Key Takeaways

- Parasites may be ectoparasitic or endoparasitic in nature.
- All of the pediculoses are considered ectoparasites.
- All helminthic infestations are considered endoparasites.
- The treatment of ectoparasites usually involves treatment with a topical antiparasitic drug.

Quiz

1. What is the major source of an infestation with tapeworms?
   a. Tainted water
   b. Unwashed vegetables
   c. Undercooked meat
   d. Eggs

Answer: c. The main source of a tapeworm infestation is eating of undercooked meat.

2. What is the most common manifestation of a tapeworm infestation?
   a. CNS findings
   b. Anemia
   c. Abdominal pain
   d. Tapeworm segments in feces

Answer: d. Most patients have no particular symptoms but may notice tapeworm segments in their stool. The other findings are less common.

3. What is the animal source seen in the disease called cysticercosis?
   a. Pork
   b. Beef
   c. Sheep
   d. Dogs

Answer: a. Cysticercosis is the name given to the pork tapeworm.

4. What tertiary complication is not caused by an ascaris infection?
   a. Pancreatitis
   b. Bowel obstruction
   c. Hepatitis
   d. Cholecystitis

Answer: c. Each of these can be caused by a tertiary ascaris infection except for hepatitis.

5. What is the most accurate diagnostic test for patients with ascariasis?
   a. Antibody testing of the blood
   b. Antigen testing of the blood
   c. Antigen testing of the stool
   d. direct visualization

Answer: d. Direct visualization of the stool sample will show evidence of the eggs or live worms in the stool.

6. How is filariasis commonly spread to humans?
    a. Eating raw fish
    b. Getting bit by a blackfly or mosquito
    c. Drinking tainted water
    d. Touching surfaces containing human feces

Answer: b. The vector for the disease involves getting bit or stung by a mosquito or the blackfly that is infected with the larvae.

7. Which of the following parasitic infection is considered an ectoparasite?
    a. Filariasis
    b. Scabies
    c. Cestodiasis
    d. Ascariasis

Answer: b. Of the above parasitic choices, only scabies is an ectoparasite. The other choices are called endoparasites.

8. Why is crusted scabies more contagious than regular scabies?
    a. The organism is closer to the skin surface.
    b. The organism is more pathogenic.
    c. The organism causes a greater immune response.
    d. There are millions of organisms versus just a few in regular scabies.

Answer: d. Only about 10-15 scabies mites are seen in regular scabies, while there are millions of organisms seen in crusted scabies, increasing the contagiousness of the disease.

9. Which is not considered one of the top three infectious skin disorders in children?
    a. Impetigo
    b. Erysipelas
    c. Scabies
    d. Ringworm

Answer: b. Erysipelas is seen more often in adults.

10. Which of the following symptoms is most common in patients with pediculosis capitis?
    a. Itching
    b. Fever
    c. Lymphadenopathy
    d. Local pain

Answer: a. Most patients who are symptomatic only get itching. Rarely, the other symptoms/signs can be seen with local pain stemming from a secondary bacterial infection.

Chapter 7: Antibiotics and Antiviral Agents

In this chapter, the topic will be antimicrobial medications, known as antibiotics, and antiviral drugs. There are dozens of antibiotics that vary according to their mechanism of action on different bacterial organisms. Some antibiotics are bactericidal and kill bacteria outright, while others are bacteriostatic, meaning that they stop the growth of bacteria and require an intact immune system to be functional against bacterial infections. Drugs that act against viruses mainly attack an element of the life cycle of viruses, while there are a select few that enhance the immune system's response against viral organisms.

Using Antibiotics in Medicine

Antibiotics have, as their purpose, the ability to prevent and treat bacterial infections, with different antibiotics acting on different types of bacterial species. A few antibiotics can kill protozoal and bacterial species equally (especially metronidazole). Whenever the exact organism is unknown, a broad-spectrum antibiotic is used to treat the infection while cultures of the stool, blood, or skin lesions are pending. Many gastroenterological infections are treated with metronidazole and another antibiotic to cover as many possible enteric pathogens as possible.

Other antibiotics can be used empirically for suspected bacterial lung infections, sinusitis, skin infections, meningitis, septicemia, or genitourinary infections that are based on the most probable causative organism. When the pathogen has been identified by culture and sensitivities, a more targeted antibiotic is used. Using cultures and sensitivities decreases the risk of antibiotic resistances.

Sensitivities involves growing the pathogen responsible for the infection in a Petri dish in the presence of a variety of discs impregnated with antibiotics. If the bacterial pathogen doesn't grow in the vicinity of the disc, it is said to be "sensitive" to the antibiotic, making it a good antibacterial choice. Culture and sensitivities are routinely performed together to save time when selecting the correct antibiotic choice. The antibiotic with the greatest clearing around the disc will be used as the antibiotic of choice.

Antibiotics can be used to prevent infections and often given to patients who have a compromised immune system and at high-risk for bacterial infections, such as HIV patients, patients on immunosuppressive medications (such as transplant patients), and cancer patients. Patients having surgery are often given preventative antibiotics at the time of surgery to prevent a surgical infection. Dental antibiotic prophylaxis is used to prevent infective endocarditis in patients with valvular disease who might get the infection secondary to bacteremia caused by dental procedures. Patients who have neutropenia are often placed on antibiotics as a prophylactic measure (although it will only prevent bacterial infections, not viral infections).

Antibiotics can be given orally, intravenously, intramuscularly, or topically, in the form of ear drops, eye drops, or topical skin preparations. Acne and cellulitis are often treated with topical antibiotics placed on the skin at the site of the infection. Bacitracin (mupirocin) is one antibiotic that is only topical and used to treat skin and certain nasal infections caused by S. aureus. Bacitracin has no systemic activity, which makes it fairly safe to give with limited allergic potential.

Topical antibiotics like Neosporin can also be used after surgery on surgical wounds to prevent post-operative infections. The biggest risk of this practice is that some of the antibiotic can get into the system (through the surgical incision) in unpredictable ways and cause a hypersensitivity reaction, systemic toxicity, or contact dermatitis (localized allergic rash) where the antibiotic was applied.

All antibiotics are screened for adverse effects before being used on the public. Most antibiotics are completely safe but some will have adverse side effects. Certain antibiotics, for example Penicillin, may cause a hypersensitivity or anaphylactic reaction. Other drugs carry a risk of photosensitivity, or the presence of a rash on sun-exposed areas of the body. The tetracycline class of antibiotics cause "photodermatitis" or extreme sunburns when patients taking them are exposed to the sun.

Common side-effects for all antibiotics include diarrhea, caused by oral or parenteral antibiotics that destroy healthy bacterial flora in the gut, resulting in an overgrowth of more resistant pathogenic flora, such as Clostridium difficile. Women who take systemic antibiotics are especially prone to getting candida yeast infections of the vagina for the same reason. Rarely, the combined use of a quinolone and a corticosteroid (parenterally or orally) can cause tendon ruptures.

There are a few studies suggesting that antibiotics might make birth control pills less effective, while there are other studies that have not shown this to be the case. It is possible that nausea, vomiting, or diarrhea from oral antibiotics might adversely affect the absorption of ethinyl estradiol in the GI tract, lowering the effective dose. For this reason, women with known menstrual irregularities should use a backup method of birth control during and for a week after taking an antibiotic for any reason.

There are some antibiotics that have a decreased effectiveness or side effects if taken along with alcohol. Antibiotics like metronidazole, tinidazole, cephamandole, and latamoxef will cause a disulfiram-like reaction with alcohol, resulting in shortness of breath, nausea, and vomiting.

Certain infectious diseases require more than one antibiotic for effective treatment. This is called "combination therapy" and is used for conditions like tuberculosis that have a high inherent potential for resistances. The combined use of more than one antibiotic has a synergistic effect, maximizing the chance of eliminating the infection.

Another condition that should be treated with combined antibiotic therapy is methicillin-resistant Staphylococcus aureus (MRSA). It is often treated with a combination of rifampin and fusidic acid (although there are still a few single antibiotics that cover for MRSA, such as vancomycin and mupirocin ointment).

In rare cases, antibiotics should not be given together because the different antibiotics antagonize one another. An example of this is tetracycline or chloramphenicol, both of which antagonize aminoglycosides and penicillin drugs. Any antibiotic that is bacteriostatic may be antagonistic to a bactericidal antibiotic.

Classes of Antibiotics

Antibiotics come from a wide range of classes based on their spectrum of activity, similar chemical structure, or similar mechanism of action. There are antibiotics that destroy the cell wall of bacteria (such as penicillin drugs and cephalosporins), those that block bacterial enzymes (such as sulfonamides, quinolones, and rifampin), and those that destroy the bacterial cell membrane (such as polymyxin). These are all bactericidal because they kill the bacterial organisms outright.

The macrolides, tetracycline antibiotics, and lincosamides are considered bacteriostatic and need a competent immune system to be effective. These block protein synthesis in the microorganism so the organism can't grow and divide effectively.

The following is a list of antibiotic classes and the way they act against microorganisms:

- **Aminoglycosides.** These include drugs like gentamycin, neomycin, tobramycin, amikacin, and paromomycin. These mainly kill Gram-negative bacteria, such as Escherichia coli, Klebsiella, and Pseudomonas aeruginosa. They cannot be given orally (must be IV) and can cause hearing loss, renal toxicity, or vertigo in high doses. They bind to a ribosomal subunit on bacteria, preventing accurate translation so no protein synthesis can happen.
- **Carbapenems.** These include imipenem/cilastin, ertapenem, and meropenem. They are bactericidal for both Gram-positive and Gram-negative organisms, making them useful as broad-spectrum antibiotics when the type of organism isn't known yet. They act by inhibiting cell wall synthesis, making them bactericidal.
- **First Generation Cephalosporins.** These include cefadroxil, cefalexin, and cefazolin, which are mainly bactericidal against Gram-positive organisms. They block the synthesis of the peptidoglycan cell wall of the bacterial organisms. These can be used to treat streptococcal pharyngitis, skin infections, and soft tissue infections. They are not good choices for acute otitis media because of resistances. They have good Gram-positive cocci coverage for Streptococcus and Staphylococcus.
- **Second Generation Cephalosporins.** These include ceprozil, cefuroxime, and cefaclor, which have less Gram-positive organism coverage and better Gram-negative coverage. The main side effects include GI upset and allergic reactions. They act by blocking the synthesis of the peptidoglycan cell wall of bacterial organisms. The major indications include respiratory tract infections, acute sinusitis, and otitis media.
- **Third Generation Cephalosporins.** They include cefotaxime, ceftazidime, cefdinir, and cefpodoxime, which have good Gram-positive coverage and good Gram-negative coverage with the exception of Pseudomonas. They may not cover well for Mycoplasma or Chlamydia. Like other beta-lactam drugs, they block the synthesis of the bacterial cell wall, and have GI upset or allergic reactions as major side effects.
- **Fourth Generation Cephalosporins.** This includes cefepime, which provides good pseudomonas coverage. It is bactericidal and eliminates the ability of the bacterium to make a cell wall.
- **Fifth Generation Cephalosporins.** This is basically just ceftobiprole and ceftaroline fosamil. They provide good coverage against MRSA and act similar to other cephalosporins with the same possible side effects.
- **Glycopeptides.** These include teicoplanin, vancomycin, and dalbavancin. They have activity against both anaerobes and aerobes, including most Gram-positive organisms, including MRSA. Oral vancomycin is used to treat colitis from Clostridium difficile. They are bactericidal through inhibiting cell wall synthesis.
- **Lincosamides.** These are bacteriostatic antibiotics, including clindamycin and lincomycin, which are good for extremely complicated staphylococcal infections, streptococcal infections, and pneumococcal infections in patients who are allergic to penicillin. They also act against anaerobes. One major side effect is pseudomembranous colitis secondary to Clostridium difficile overgrowth. They bind to the 50S subunit on ribosomal transfer RNA, blocking the synthesis of proteins by the bacterial species.
- **Lincopeptide.** This includes daptomycin, which acts against Gram-positive organisms but doesn't work well for pneumonia because surfactant in the lungs inhibits its action. It causes

depolarization of the cell membrane of the bacteria so there is a lack of nucleic acid and protein synthesis.

- **Macrolides.** This is a large group that includes azithromycin, clarithromycin, erythromycin, and roxithromycin. They act against streptococcal organisms, mycoplasma, syphilis, Lyme disease, pneumonias, pelvic infection in pregnancy, Legionella pneumophila, Bordetella pertussis, Corynebacterium diphtheriae, Campylobacter jejuni, and upper respiratory reactions. They can cause GI upset, prolonged QT interval, and possible hearing loss at high doses. They work by blocking bacterial protein synthesis by binding to a subunit on the bacterial ribosome. These are bacteriostatic.
- **Monobactams.** This includes aztreonam, which is effective against Gram-negative bacteria. It has a similar mode of action as all bactericidal beta-lactams and kills bacteria by disrupting cell wall synthesis.
- **Nitrofurans.** This includes nitrofurantoin, which is used exclusively for urinary tract infections. A less common antibiotic of this class is furazolidone, which is used for protozoal or bacterial GI tract infections.
- **Oxazolidinones.** These are bacteriostatic antibiotics, such as linezolid and posizolid. They act against vancomycin-resistant Staphylococcal aureus infections. The major side effects are thrombocytopenia, serotonin syndrome, or peripheral neuropathy. They block a step in protein synthesis so the organism can no longer grow effectively.
- **Penicillins.** This is a large group of antibiotics, including amoxicillin, carbenicillin, ampicillin, dicloxacillin, nafcillin, methicillin, mezlocillin, and cloxacillin. They are bactericidal and effective against streptococcal infections, Lyme disease, and syphilis. The major side effects are anaphylactic reactions and GI disturbances. They act by blocking the synthesis of the bacterial cell wall.
- **Polypeptides.** This includes just bacitracin, polymyxin B, and colistin, which are used topically or inhaled. They are bactericidal antibiotics with slightly different modes of action. Bacitracin blocks isoprenyl pyrophosphate, which is necessary for the building of the cell wall, while the others have an adverse effect on the outer cell membrane, causing a displacement of counterions in the membrane which dissolves the membrane. There can be nervous system and renal damage when given intravenously, this is rarely done unless there is a multidrug resistance in the infection.
- **Quinolones or Fluoroquinolones.** This includes ciprofloxacin, levofloxacin, lomefloxacin, ofloxacin, norfloxacin, and a few less commonly-used bactericidal drugs. They are often used for bacterial prostatitis, gonorrhea, mycoplasma, bacterial diarrheal illnesses, pneumonia, and UTIs. Nausea is uncommon, while rare tendon rupture can occur when these are mixed with concurrent corticosteroid use. They work by blocking the bacterial DNA gyrase enzyme or the topoisomerase IV enzyme, which effectively blocks replication and transcription of DNA.
- **Sulfonamides.** These are bacteriostatic antibiotics that include silver sulfadiazine, sulfacetamide, sulfasalazine, sulfisoxazole, and trimethoprim-sulfamethoxazole. They are primarily used for UTIs and Pneumocystis carinii (prophylaxis and treatment) but some topical forms (like sulfacetamide and silver sulfadiazine) are used for skin or eye infections. Side effects include nausea and vomiting, allergic skin rashes, leukopenia, photodermatitis, and kidney dysfunction. They inhibit the folate synthesis through competitive inhibition of dihydropteroate synthetase. Without folate, the cell can't divide and growth is inhibited.
- **Tetracyclines.** This include tetracycline, doxycycline, minocycline, and a few others. These are bacteriostatic drugs that are effective against syphilis, mycoplasma, rickettsia, malaria, chlamydia, and Lyme disease. They cause side effects that include photosensitivity, teeth

staining in kids, GI distress, and potential fetal toxicity in pregnancy. They work by binding the complex of aminoacyl-tRNA and mRNA, inhibiting the translation process.

- **Anti-Mycobacterial Drugs.** These will fight off mycobacterial species, such a tuberculosis and leprosy, and are bactericidal. They include things like dapsone, clofazimine, cycloserine, ethambutol, ethionamide, isoniazid, streptomycin, and rifampicin. Some are effective against tuberculosis, while others act more against leprosy. They act on different parts of the cell, including several different ways to block protein synthesis.
- **Miscellaneous Antibiotics.** There are several antibiotics that have no particular classification. These include chloramphenicol, fosfomycin, mupirocin, arsphenamine, metronidazole, and fusidic acid. They have varying mechanisms of action and used for many diseases. Metronidazole, for example, is used for amoebiasis, trichomoniasis, and giardiasis, and anaerobic bacteria infections, such as Bacteroides fragilis, Clostridium difficile, and bacterial vaginosis. It can cause discolored urine, headache, and a disulfiram-like interaction with alcohol. It acts by making toxic free radicals that destroy bacterial DNA and proteins. Mupirocin goes by the brand name of Bactroban and is a topical ointment for impetigo and the prevention of infection in wound care. It blocks protein synthesis by blocking t-RNA synthetase.

Antiviral Drugs

Antiviral drugs are a type of medication that specifically targets viral infections. There are broad-spectrum antiviral drugs and narrow-spectrum antiviral drugs. One of the biggest differences between antiviral agents and antibacterial drugs is that there is no antiviral agent that will kill the particle. The drug will only block the growth and development of the virus, requiring a competent immune system to kill the organism.

Antiviral medications fall under the classification of antimicrobial agents, which includes other antimicrobial agents, such as antibiotics, antifungal drugs, and antiparasitic drugs. Most antiviral drugs are extremely safe for the host as they act on microorganisms that are very different from the host cells which limits side effects. Antiviral drugs are not the same as viricides, which are not considered medications but act outside the body to destroy or deactivate viral particles. There are natural antiviral agents that are produced by certain plants. One example of this is the eucalyptus plant, which secretes an antiviral agent.

Most of the antiviral drugs out there are effective against only a few types of viruses. Viruses that have known antiviral agents that act against them include the HIV virus, influenza A, influenza B, hepatitis C, hepatitis B, and herpesviruses. Most other viruses cannot be killed with antiviral agents.

The challenge is to discover antiviral drugs that can adversely affect viral growth without harming the human host. This is difficult because the viral particle is often found inside the host cell so the medication must penetrate the cell to have activity against the viral particle.

Another challenge is the fact that viruses are very different from one another and they change their genomes often. What works for one type of virus will not work for another type of virus. Even so, research has effectively found antiviral medications that successfully attack several of the most severe viruses that infect humans, particularly HIV disease and hepatis B/C infections.

The first antiviral drugs were used against herpes viruses and were developed in the 1960s. Cultures of infected cells were mixed with different agents until, by trial-and-error, safe drugs were found that didn't have a major effect on the host cells. No one at that time understood how viruses worked and there was no genetic sequencing going on at that time. Nevertheless, several good drugs were developed.

Antiviral drugs attempt to tackle the different aspects of the viral life cycle, including its host attachment, release of viral genes into the host, replication inside the host, viral assembly after replication of the genome, and release of new viral particles.

When identifying a good antiviral agent, researchers must target certain aspects of the life cycle of the virus without harming the host cell. Ideally, an antiviral should cover for many strains of a virus so that a mutation won't render the antiviral agent ineffective. The best antiviral agent should cover against many different species of viral particles, such as all the viruses of the same family, giving the drug broad coverage.

In order for a virus to become infective, the viral particle must inject its DNA or RNA into the host cell, or must enter the cell. Viruses that contain a lipid covering need to first fuse this covering with the target cell or must form a vesicle in which to get into the cell. It is after this that the virus uncoats. There can be drugs made that bind to the virus-associated protein on the cell so the virus particle has no protein available to bind to it. This type of antiviral drug includes things like anti-VAP antibody drugs or natural ligands for the receptor. VAP anti-idiotypic antibodies would also theoretically be successful.

When this is applied to treating the HIV virus, drugs are currently being developed that specifically block the receptors on the CD4+ cells, which are the main cells of entry for the HIV virus and the cells targeted for destruction by the HIV virus. So far, efforts at interfering with the HIV-binding site on the CD4+ cell haven't effectively stopped the infection, but there are promising ongoing research efforts.

Other efforts have attempted to block the entry of HIV cells into T helper cells by blocking the step where the virus fuses with the eukaryotic cell. One biomimetic peptide that will do this is being used on HIV patients now, under the brand name of Fuzeon. It is believed to stop the spread of infection inside an infected patient and reduce the spread of the virus from person-to-person. One other advantage of this type of drug is that it targets the life cycle of the virus before it has a chance to mutate into a different form.

There are also drugs that adversely affect or block the uncoating process of a viral particle. Both amantadine and rimantadine are drugs that act directly on the penetration and uncoating process of the influenza virus, which also affects the virus before it has a chance to mutate.

There are antiviral drugs that are in the works that act to block the synthesis of new viral particles after the virus has already uncoated and invaded the cell. One way this works is to have nucleotide or nucleoside analogues that simulate normal building blocks of RNA or DNA. They bind to the transcriptase enzyme of the virus and inhibit it from making a new viral genome. The reverse transcriptase inhibitors in use today work in this way and don't affect human cells because they use a "normal" transcriptase. This is basic mechanism of acyclovir, used to treat the herpesvirus, and zidovudine (AZT), which is used to treat HIV disease.

Still another drug, lamivudine, has been approved by the Food and Drug Administration to treat hepatitis B, which also makes use of a reverse transcriptase enzyme as part of its infectious process. This drug binds to the hepatitis B reverse transcriptase molecule, preventing it from turning RNA into DNA inside the host cell.

Another HIV drug being researched is a drug that acts on RNase H, which is the part of the reverse transcriptase molecule that breaks off the newly synthesized DNA molecule from the viral RNA template. This is being researched for more than just the HIV virus and will have wide applications should it be approved.

Another target is the integrase molecule, which takes the DNA synthesized by the reverse transcriptase and integrates it into the human genome. This could work against viruses that depend on this step as part of their process of replication inside the host cell.

After the DNA gets incorporated into the host genome (in the infected cell), it makes a lot of mRNA that then synthesizes the necessary viral proteins to make new virus particles. This is initiated by certain transcription factors that need to be activated to make the mRNA in the first place. There are antiviral drugs being evaluated that block the attachment of these transcription factors to the viral DNA segment.

There is a brand-new type of drug that is based on "antisense" segments. These are the complementary strands to crucial parts of the viral genome. If the antisense segment is blocked with a drug, the viral genome cannot be replicated. There is one drug available that does this, called fomivirsin, which treats viral eye infections in patients with HIV disease (who frequently get cytomegalovirus infections of the eye).

Antiviral agents can be developed that are based on ribozymes, which are the enzymes that normally cut the viral genome at a specific place. Ribozymes are necessary in the manufacturing of a new viral particle. There are ribozyme-based drugs being studied for hepatitis A and HIV but there are no currently-available drugs for this.

Protease inhibitors exist that act as antiviral agents. Viruses often use certain proteases to break apart long strands of proteins into their proper length. HIV is one of the viruses that uses this type of enzyme. This is why a lot of research has been done to find drugs that can block this process in HIV disease. There are protease inhibitors on the market that are effective against the HIV virus.

There is also the assembly and release phases of the lifecycle to consider. The drug known as rifampicin acts to block the assembly of the virus particles. Other drugs, such as Relenza (zanamivir) and Tamiflu (oseltamivir) act against influenza by blocking neuraminidase, an enzyme found on the surface of the influenza virus particle that is necessary for its ability to release living new particles from the infected host cell.

Another way of approaching an antiviral drug is to stimulate the immune system to kill the virus more effectively rather than actually attacking the virus particle itself. The class of medications that do this the best are called "interferons". They block the synthesis of the virus in an infected cell. Drugs that do this are effective against both hepatitis B and hepatitis C, including interferon alpha. Other interferon drugs are being considered as good antiviral agents.

Monoclonal antibodies are another way of fighting viral infections. The process involves finding the right protein on the virus particle and making a great deal of antibodies against that specific protein. This can be given to a human host and act similar to the antibodies they would create, but would produce them faster than a human cell makes antibodies. This type of drug is being used to treat respiratory syncytial virus.

Common Antiviral Drugs

There aren't as many antiviral drugs as there are antibiotic drugs, although there is much research in the field directed at stopping the synthesis of new viral particle and halting the process of viral replication. There are often-used antivirals against influenza, hepatitis, herpesvirus, and HIV disease.

Amantadine

This is marketed as Symmetrel, a drug for both Parkinson's disease and influenza A. It is related to the antiviral drug rimantadine. Unfortunately, virtually 100 percent of the latest strains of influenza are resistant to amantadine so it is no longer recommended for routine use in the management of influenza diseases. Recent studies have also indicated that it is not effective for the prevention of influenza.

Relenza (zanamivir)

Zanamivir is marketed as Relenza and is used to treat both influenza A and influenza B. It is a neuraminidase inhibitor, first approved in 1999 in the US after being first licensed for use in other parts of the world in 1990. It is used for the prevention and treatment of these diseases. There have been a few cases resistances but it is effective as an inhaled powder for most cases of influenza A/B. It shortens the course of the disease by about a day so it isn't necessarily helpful in healthy patients. It doesn't seem to decrease the risk of hospitalizations or secondary complications.

Tamiflu (oseltamivir phosphate)

Oseltamivir is sold under the trade name of Tamiflu, which is used to treat and prevent influenza A and influenza B. It is used within the first 48 hours of symptoms and as a preventative in high risk patients only. It is a liquid or pill treatment. It doesn't seem to decrease the hospitalization rate or the risk of complications in influenza. However, tt does seem to be an effective preventative treatment. It is used to treat influenza in pregnancy and is a neuraminidase inhibitor. The risk versus benefit is controversial as there are side effects in taking the drug and it is expensive.

Rapivab (peramivir)

Peramivir is an antiviral drug and a neuraminidase inhibitor used to treat influenza. It blocks the release of newly made virus particles from infected cells. It is used as an IV drug for serious cases of influenza. It has been approved for use in influenza since 2014. It is the only intravenous option for the treatment of the swine flu.

Adefovir

Adefovir is used specifically to treat chronic hepatitis B infections. Its function is as a reverse transcriptase inhibitor and can also be used for herpes simplex virus infections (less frequently). It is ineffective as a treatment for HIV disease. It is reserved for hepatitis B patients who have elevated ALT or have histological evidence of active chronic hepatitis. While resistances can develop, it takes a period of time before it is evident so it can control the disease in the meantime.

Famciclovir

This drug is a guanosine analogue for the treatment of herpes zoster. It is the prodrug of the penciclovir drug with good oral bioavailability and is marketed as Famvir. It has been in use since 1994 with generic drugs available since 2007. It can also be used for cold sores and herpes simplex type II in immunocompetent patients. It can be used in HIV patients to treat recurrent herpes simplex virus infections. When given to a first-time herpes simplex patient, it will prevent outbreaks of recurrent infections—superior to valaciclovir-treated patients and acyclovir-treated patients.

Interferon

There is a variety of interferon drugs used as signaling proteins released by host cells after exposure to many types of pathogens. Virus-infected cells release interferon in order to enhance the anti-viral activity of nearby cells. Interferon is a type of cytokine used to communicate information from one cell to another. The drug can interfere with the replication of viruses and can activate macrophages and NK cells by causing an increase in MCH antigens. There are about twenty interferons in the body, divided into three major classes.

Type I interferons are made when the body recognizes a viral invasion, preventing viral replication. Interferon-alpha used to treat hepatitis B and hepatitis C infections and interferon-beta is used to treat multiple sclerosis. Type II interferon is "immune interferon" released by T helper cells. It is used in the management of multiple sclerosis. Interferon type III is more recently identified as playing a role in virus infections.

Acyclovir and Valacyclovir

Both of these drugs are used primarily for the treatment of herpes simplex virus infections (but can be used in chickenpox and shingles outbreaks, and in both CMV and Epstein-Barr virus infections). They can be applied to the skin, taken orally, or injected. The main side effects are diarrhea and nausea with the only possible severe side effects being thrombocytopenia and kidney insufficiency. They are extremely inexpensive and can be used as preventative or treatment of herpesvirus infections.

Complex herpes simplex viral diseases can be treated with these medications, including neonatal herpes, herpes simplex labialis disease (cold sores), chickenpox in the immunosuppressed patient, herpes blepharitis, and herpes simplex encephalitis. It is not effective in treating infectious mononucleosis because of the Epstein-Barr virus. It will not prevent HIV transmission but can slow the disease progression of HIV in patients not on anti-retroviral therapy for HIV disease.

Key Takeaways

- Antimicrobial agents include antibiotics, which can be bactericidal or bacteriostatic drugs.
- All antiviral drugs interfere with viral activity but don't kill the virus directly.
- There can be resistances in both antiviral drugs and antibiotics.
- There are many antibiotic drugs but only a few antiviral drugs that act on a select few viral infections.
- Antiviral drugs exist for HIV disease, influenza, hepatitis B, hepatitis C, and herpesvirus infections.

Quiz

1. Which antibiotic is well-known to destroy protozoa as well as bacteria?
   a. Ciprofloxacin
   b. Clindamycin
   c. Metronidazole
   d. Amoxicillin/clavulanate

Answer: c. Metronidazole can destroy both bacterial organisms and protozoal species.

2. What is the main advantage of doing antibiotic sensitivities?
   a. There is no need to do antibiotic sensitivities.
   b. Sensitivities indicate if the bacteria are able to be controlled by the antibiotic.
   c. Sensitivities indicate if more than one antibiotic is necessary.
   d. Sensitivities indicate if the antibiotic is bactericidal or bacteriostatic.

Answer: b. Sensitivities indicate if the bacteria are able to be controlled by the antibiotic. It may be bacteriostatic or bactericidal in nature.

3. Which patient is least likely to be immunosuppressed and would least likely need prophylactic antibiotics?
   a. The patient with an organ transplant
   b. The patient with HIV disease
   c. The patient with cancer on chemotherapy
   d. The patient with diabetes mellitus

Answer: d. Each of these types of patients is immunosuppressed to such a degree that they would need prophylactic antibiotics except for the diabetic patient, who is less immunosuppressed than the other choices.

4. Which antimicrobial agent will not have a disulfiram-like reaction when taken with alcohol?
   a. Metronidazole
   b. Tinidazole

c. Cephamandole

d. Ciprofloxacin

Answer: d. Each of the choices will cause a disulfiram-like reaction when taken with alcohol except for ciprofloxacin.

5. Which infectious disease is most likely to require combination therapy because of a high rate of resistances?

   a. Tuberculosis

   b. Pertussis

   c. Streptococcal pharyngitis

   d. Erysipelas

Answer: a. Of the above choices, tuberculosis has a high rate of resistances and should be treated with more than one antibiotic.

6. Which class of antibiotic can cause hearing loss when given to patients with Gram-negative infections?

   a. Tetracyclines

   b. Aminoglycosides

   c. Carbapenems

   d. Third-generation cephalosporins

Answer: b. Aminoglycosides have a high risk of hearing loss and a narrow therapeutic window so levels need to be checked to make sure the antibiotic isn't in the toxic range.

7. Which type of virus cannot be treated with an antiviral agent?

   a. Influenza A

   b. Herpesvirus

   c. Hepatitis C

   d. Rhinovirus

Answer: d. There are antiviral drugs for all of these viruses except for rhinovirus, which does not have an antiviral agent that works against it.

8. Which antiviral drugs were developed historically (in the 1960s)?

   a. Anti-hepatitis B

   b. Anti-hepatitis C

   c. Anti-herpes virus

   d. Anti-influenza

Answer: c. The first antiviral drugs were discovered by trial-and-error against the herpes virus in the 1960s. The other antiviral drugs came later.

9. Which type of antiviral drug has activity against the HIV virus?

   a. Reverse transcriptase drugs

   b. Anti-VAP antibody drugs

   c. Monoclonal antibody drugs

   d. Anti-ribosomal drugs

Answer: a. There are reverse transcriptase drugs that have activity against the HIV virus. The other types of drugs are used against other types of viruses.

10. Which antiviral drug is used specifically to treat herpes simplex infections?
    a. Valacyclovir
    b. Adefovir
    c. Peramivir
    d. Amantadine

Answer: a. Valacyclovir is used almost exclusively to treat herpes simplex type 1 and herpes simplex type 2 disease.

Chapter 8: Antifungals, Anti-Protozoal Agents, and Anti-Parasitic Agents

This chapter covers the broad topics of antifungal medications, anti-protozoal medications, and anti-parasitic medications. Antifungal drugs can be topical, intravenous, or oral. Anti-protozoal drugs are generally oral drugs and vary depending on the protozoal organism being treated. Anti-parasitic drugs can be ingested to treat helminthiasis or used externally for ectoparasitic diseases, such as scabies and pediculosis infestations.

Antifungal Drugs

There are antifungal drugs for minor fungal infections, like athlete's foot, ringworm, Candida vaginitis, certain kinds of dandruff, and fungal nail infections. There are also antifungal drugs designed to treat more serious fungal infections, including disseminated diseases, like pulmonary aspergillosis, disseminated Candidiasis, and fungal meningitis. These fungal infections are more common among immunosuppressed patients, and require IV antibiotics.

Types of antifungals include a variety of topical agents (ointments, sprays, gels, and creams that are directly applied to the area of infection), oral pills for fungal infections, and intravenous antifungals used in hospital settings for severe disease. For vaginitis, there are antifungal suppositories and vaginal pessaries used to treat the disorder. Antifungal drugs act by killing the fungal cells directly or by preventing the growth and replication of fungal cells.

Clotrimazole

Clotrimazole is a common antifungal drug used for many types of fungal diseases, including jock itch, athlete's foot, ringworm, pityriasis versicolor, diaper rash, thrush, and candida vaginitis. It is available as an oral substance or a topical agent. It is safe to take in pregnancy as a topical, however oral used during pregnancy has been less well-studied. It must be used with care in people with liver insufficiency. It is azole drug that disrupts the cell membrane, killing the fungal cell. It's been on the market since the early 1970s and is considered among the safest drugs of its type.

It is available without a prescription as a vaginal tablet and cream but needs a prescription for the throat lozenge (troche). It is one of the main treatments for vulvovaginal candidiasis, where it is used topically, and for skin infections caused by fungal organisms. It can be given as a throat lozenge for the prevention of oral candidiasis in patients who are neutropenic. It is combined with betamethasone and other glucocorticoids in the management of athlete's foot, jock itch, and ringworm (tinea corporis). The biggest problem with using this combination is that it blocks the immune response and can cause secondary skin atrophy if used for a long period of time.

Miconazole

Miconazole, also known as Monistat, is a popular drug used to treat vaginal yeast infections, as well as for the treatment of pityriasis versicolor and ring worm. It is solely used as a topical cream, ointment, or vaginal suppository. It is believed to be safe to take in pregnancy without harm to the fetus. It is an imidazole drug and stops fungal cell wall growth by inhibiting the ability of the fungus to use ergosterol as part of the cell membrane. It's been in use since 1971 and is considered a safe and effective drug that is also inexpensive.

The main uses of miconazole include the management of ringworm, jock itch, athlete's foot, oral thrush, vaginal yeast infections, and angular cheilitis. It is used in newborn thrush as well. It can interact with other drugs if allowed to absorb through the GI tract or vaginal lining, including anticoagulants, phenytoin, statin drugs, atypical antipsychotics, cyclosporin, and terbinafine.

Terbinafine

Terbinafine is marketed as Lamisil. It is used to treat fungal nail infections, pityriasis versicolor, jock itch, and ringworm. It can be taken orally or topically but must be taken orally to treat onychomycosis. The main side effects include allergies and liver dysfunction. It is not recommended in pregnancy. Its mechanism of action involves inhibiting sterol production of fungi, making it a fungicidal drug. It has been in use since the middle of the 1990s and is generally considered a safe and effective drug.

Terbinafine is used as a treatment for ringworm, jock itch, and athlete's foot, and seems to work in half the time as other topical drugs. Oral terbinafine is used to treat onychomycosis but carries a risk of hepatotoxicity when taken orally. For this reason, periodic liver tests are recommended to make sure that the liver is not adversely affected. It can also exacerbate systemic lupus erythematosus symptoms.

Fluconazole

Fluconazole is used as an antifungal drug for a variety of fungal infections, including dermatophytoses, pityriasis versicolor, blastomycosis, candidiasis, cryptococcosis, coccidioidomycosis, and histoplasmosis. It can be used orally or intravenously in patients at high risk for fungal diseases, including neutrophilic patients, premature infants, and organ transplant patients. It can cause seizures, QT prolongation, and hepatotoxicity. It has been used on the market since 1988 and is generally considered safe.

The main diseases that fluconazole is used for include Candida infections (of just about any body area) in immunocompetent people, for cryptococcal meningoencephalitis (second-line drug), and for the prevention of Candida infections in immunocompromised hosts. This is an azole drug that can result in resistances when used for a long period of time. Resistance to one azole means resistance to all other azole drugs. The overall resistance rate in Candida organisms is about seven percent.

Ketoconazole

This is an imidazole drug used to treat a variety of fungal infections, such as seborrheic dermatitis, pityriasis versicolor, paronychia (from candida), cutaneous candidiasis, and tinea infections. It can be used systemically but is not as safe as itraconazole and fluconazole. It is not used systemically for humans in many parts of the world because of a greater risk of hepatotoxicity when used systemically.

Topically, the drug ketoconazole is used for a variety of skin and mucous membrane-related dermatophytoses and candida infections (including jock itch, ringworm, and athlete's foot). It is used topically for seborrheic dermatitis (anywhere on the body). While it can be used for systemic infections, it is not a first-line drug because of poorer absorption and increased toxicity compared to other azoles.

Amphotericin B

Amphotericin B is an antifungal agent used solely for serious fungal infections. It can be used alone or with IV flucytosine for cryptococcosis, coccidioidomycosis, candidiasis, blastomycosis, and aspergillosis. It can also be used to treat leishmaniasis. It can lead to renal toxicity, fever, headaches, and chills when given. Allergies to the drug, myocarditis, and hypokalemia can come from using the drug. The lipid form has fewer side effects. It interferes with the cell membrane synthesis in fungal organisms, making it fungicidal. It is safe in pregnancy.

Because of the severe side effects associated with taking Amphotericin B, it is not a first line drug unless the patient is very ill or immunosuppressed. It is first-line for aspergillosis, systemic candidiasis, cryptococcal meningitis, and mucormycosis infections. It has been used for more than 50 years successfully because of a low risk of resistance. Several protozoal infections can be treated with amphotericin B, including visceral leishmaniasis and amoebic infections.

The drug alone isn't soluble at human pH levels so it is altered to make it bioavailable as an IV drug. There is an amphotericin B deoxycholate form that has a lot of side effects so it isn't used as often as other types. Lipid forms (liposomal forms) have less renal toxicity so they are preferred over conventional amphotericin. Liposomal amphotericin B is used for CNS fungal infections because of better CNS penetration. There are several types of lipid-soluble amphotericin B preparations that can be used.

Anti-Protozoal Drugs

Antiprotozoal drugs are a group of medications used to treat different types of protozoal infections, including intestinal and blood-based infections. There is a special class of medications used to treat malaria called antimalarial drugs. Symptoms treated in malarial disease include myalgias, nausea/vomiting, diarrhea, headache, sweating, chills, and fever. In severe cases, there can be such overwhelming symptoms that the patient dies within 24 hours of infection onset.

There are antiprotozoal drugs used to treat giardiasis, which is an intestinal infection usually contracted by drinking contaminated water and eating contaminated food. The main symptom is diarrhea but there can be other GI symptoms, such as abdominal pain and bloating.

The STD trichomoniasis is a protozoal infection passed via sexual contact. It can cause yellow vaginal discharge and vaginal itching in females and purulent urethral discharge/dysuria in males. There are specific antiprotozoal drugs used to treat this type of infection.

Antimalarial Drugs

Antimalarial drugs are collectively known as antimalarials, which can be used for the prevention or treatment of malaria. It is used for patients with known malaria, to prevent malaria in visitors to malaria-endemic areas of the world, and to treat groups of patients in endemic areas (routine prevention). The treatment of malaria should be done on confirmed cases only with combination therapy, which reduces resistances and decreases side effects.

Quinine is the oldest agent used for treating malaria. It comes from the bark of the cinchona tree and is actually a related group of drugs. The drug is an alkaloid that builds up in the food vacuoles of Plasmodium falciparum (the main cause of malaria). It is used in places where there are resistances to other malarial drugs. It is used for people returning from endemic areas where exposure to malaria is expected. It is often combined with clindamycin, tetracycline, or doxycycline. It can be given orally, intravenously, and intramuscularly.

There is a major side effect to using quinine, called cinchonism. It leads to hearing impairment with tinnitus, vertigo, and GI symptoms. It impairs the function of the eighth cranial nerve and can cause confusion, acute delirium, and coma. It can cause hypoglycemia in therapeutic doses by stimulating the secretion of insulin. Overdose can lead to acute renal failure and respiratory failure, leading to death.

The two most common quinine-related drugs for malaria include quinidine and Quinimax. Quinimax uses a combination of alkaloids, including quinidine, quinine, cinchonidine, and cinchoine. It uses several alkaloids for synergism and better effectiveness than just one alkaloid drug. Quinidine alone is reserved for serious malaria cases.

Chloroquine was once the most widely-used antimalarial drug and is the cheapest/safest drug for malaria. The biggest problem is resistances, which makes it more effective when used with other malaria drugs. The mechanism of action against malaria is unknown. It also treats the inflammation and fever present with P. vivax infections. It is considerably safe when used in pregnancy, making it a first-line drug in pregnant patients. A major side effect is itching.

The drug amodiaquine is similar to chloroquine and is preferred over chloroquine because of less associated itching. It is combined with artesunate (as an artemisinin combination therapy). It is given over three days like chloroquine but does carry a risk of hepatotoxicity and blood disorders when given.

Pyrimethamine is used to treat chloroquine-resistant malaria when combined with sulfadoxine. It stops all malarial DNA replication, cell division, and reproduction by blocking the synthesis of pyrimidines and purines. It is only used when combined with a sulfonamide.

Proguanil is a biguanide, which is a synthetic derivative of pyrimidine. It has been in use since 1945. It gets converted to cycloguanil that blocks the dihydrofolate reductase enzyme in the malarial organism. It cannot be used as a preventative treatment for relapse and isn't recommended for acute infection. When combined with atovaquone or chloroquine, it can be used as a prophylactic agent.

Sulfadoxine and sulfamethoxypyridazine are both sulfonamides that block the dihydropteroate synthetase enzyme in the malarial organism. They compete with PABA and act to kill the organism in its asexual cycle. When administered alone they aren't effective but when combined with pyrimethamine, they can act synergistically to kill the malarial strains. They aren't recommended as prophylactic agents because of skin-related side effects but are used for acute disease states.

Mefloquine is related to quinine and was used as a protectant against malaria in the Vietnam war. It is able to kill the malarial parasite by damaging the parasite's food vacuoles. It is used to prevent malaria in areas where there are a lot of resistances and is used for both the prevention and treatment of malaria. It is usually mixed with Artesunate. It is used in pregnant patients in all trimesters of the pregnancy. It has typical side effects with the addition of psychiatric side effects and a high degree of cardiovascular side effects (especially sinus arrhythmias). Because of its cardiac and psychiatric side effects, it should be reserved for use for only six months at a time.

Atovaquone is combined with proguanil under the trade name of Malarone. It is used as prophylaxis for travelers to malaria-prone parts of the world. It is sometimes used to treat malaria in developed countries.

Primaquine is used to treat all kinds of malarial diseases, killing the organism in various parts of the life cycle. It can cure both relapsing and acute malaria with an unknown mechanism of action. It occasionally must be used as a part of combination therapy for malaria.

There are artemisinin derivatives that come from a Chinese herb used for thousands of years in China. The drug has been isolated from the herb as an antimalarial agent. It is effective in treating all types of malaria, showing effectiveness within 1-3 days of starting the medication. Artemether is a derivative of artemisinin that can kill the malaria in just certain disease stages. Artesunate is used in combination with other drugs to treat acute malaria (being the most commonly used drug of its class). Dihydroartemisinin is a metabolite of artemisinin that has strong anti-malarial activity and is used for acute resistant cases of P. falciparum. Arteether is a derivative of dihydroartemisinin. It is used as a medication in resistant P. falciparum. Together, these drugs are widely used and the most effective way to kill malaria that is known to be resistant. Their use is highly restricted because the WHO doesn't want resistances to these drugs to develop.

Halofantrine is a new drug related to quinine that acts to kill bloodborne malarial parasites. It is effective against all forms of Plasmodium disease. It forms cytotoxic complexes with ferritoporphyrin XI that causes plasmodial membrane damage. The biggest downside of the medication is the cost; however, it does also have a high degree of cardiotoxicity. It is used with people who don't have heart disease but have severe acute malaria. It can cause severe ventricular dysrhythmias and death in some patients. It cannot be used during pregnancy.

Doxycycline is cheap and effective against malaria, despite also being an antibiotic. It is used as a preventative agent against malaria in areas of chloroquine resistance and is combined with quinine to treat resistant malaria. It cannot be used as monotherapy in acute cases because it is too slow-acting. It can't be used in children or in pregnant women because of side effects, including permanent hypoplasia of the tooth enamel. Tetracycline is similar to doxycycline but is only used in acute malaria in combination with other drugs. Clindamycin is another antibiotic used in combination with quinine to treat resistant malaria but not as a preventative medication. A major side effect is pseudomembranous colitis.

Melarsoprol

This is a drug specifically used to treat African sleeping sickness (African trypanosomiasis) in the second stage of the disease. It doesn't repair any neurological damage that has already occurred but will stop the damaging process when given intravenously. It can cause hepatotoxicity, renal toxicity, and brain dysfunction. WHO provides the drug for free in areas of the world where the disease is more common. It is the only treatment used for T. b. rhodesiense. It is highly toxic so it is only used in severe second-stage disease. There is a failure rate of about 27 percent. It results in the death of about five percent of patients who take it.

Eflornithine

This is used to treat the second stage of African sleeping sickness caused by T. b. gambiense as both a topical and injectable drug. As an IV drug, it can cause bone marrow suppression. It cannot be used in children and is provided for free by WHO in developing countries. It is commonly used in combination with oral nifurtimox to decrease the treatment time on eflornithine. It is preferred over melarsoprol because of its decreased toxicity. There are some resistances associated with the drug.

Lampit (nifurtimox)

Nifurtimox is used in combination with eflornithine for African sleeping sickness and is a second-line agent in the treatment of Chagas disease (second only to benznidazole). It is an oral drug that isn't recommended in pregnancy, liver disease, or kidney disease. It needs to be given for 30-60 days in the treatment of Chagas disease. It is used in second stage African sleeping sickness combined with melarsoprol or eflornithine.

Suramin

Suramin is used to treat both African sleeping sickness and river blindness. It is used primarily to treat first-stage trypanosomiasis via IV. There are a number of side effects with the drug that interfere with its use. It is provided for free by WHO in endemic areas. It is a second-line agent because of its serious and frequent side effects. It has also been used to treat river blindness or onchocerciasis.

Antihelminthic Drugs

These drugs represent antiparasitic drugs that get rid of helminths (parasitic worms). They stun or kill the worm and have no negative effect on the host itself. There are vermifuges (that stun the worm) and vermicides (that kill the worm). They are also called anthelmintics. Some are used in mass deworming treatments in school-aged children during epidemics of worms. Ascaricides only kill ascaris worms. The two most commonly used antihelminthic drugs are mebendazole and albendazole, which can kill threadworms, roundworms, pinworms, tapeworms, and hookworms (albendazole only). There are a number of benzimidazoles (like thiabendazole, fenbendazole, and triclabendazole) but they aren't as effective in the widest types of worms as is albendazole. Other antihelminthic drugs include ivermectin, pyrantel pamoate, and Niclosamide, which have limited usefulness. The malarial drug artemisinin is also somewhat antihelminthic in nature.

Resistance to antihelminthic drugs remains a possibility, especially in nematodes. This has spawned numerous activities that have been directed at creating newer drugs for these disorders. The problem is that some worms will develop a DNA profile that renders them non-susceptible to the drug. These worms survive the antihelminthic treatment and spread the resistance to other people, leading to a resistant strain of the organism.

Pediculosis Drugs

There are two ways to kill head lice. The first is paralyzing the head louse and the second is suffocation of the louse. The drugs that cause neurotoxicity include lindane, permethrin, malathion, and pyrethrins/piperonyl butoxide. Of these, the first-line treatment for head lice is currently permethrin (as it has the least amount of resistances and the least toxicity).

Other treatments include benzyl alcohol (a suffocation drug that is not ovicidal and is costly), ivermectin (which is partially ovicidal and inexpensive), and malathion (which is partially ovicidal, flammable, and expensive). Permethrin is not ovicidal but is inexpensive and can be given in two separate doses to kill all lice). Pyrethrins and piperonyl butoxide are used together as the trade name Rid (they act synergistically). The major downside of using lindane is that it is neurotoxic and not recommended in small adults, older people, or children, and can only be used once.

Most treatments are not reliable in destroying the eggs. Repeat treatments are necessary to get eliminate newly hatched lice after a seven-day to ten-day waiting period from the time of first treatment. There are no single-use anti-lice treatments. There is a new drug called Spinosad that paralysis the louse and is effective in treating 93 percent of cases with one treatment (versus just 63 percent eradication with permethrin). It is not widely used. Ivermectin is oral and is not FDA-approved for treating pediculosis. It is taken for up to two weeks and has a 95 percent eradication rate.

There are fewer choices out there for the treatment of scabies. The first-line treatment for the past twenty years is permethrin 5 percent cream. It is applied to the entire body from the neck down and kept on for 8-14 hours before washing it off, and repeated in one week. Itching will be present for two weeks even if the drug is effective. Another treatment is oral ivermectin, given once and again in fourteen days but Is costlier to use. Sheets and clothing need to be washed and dried on hot heat or kept in isolation in a plastic bag for 72 hours.

Crusted scabies is harder to treat than uncomplicated scabies. Treatment that is recommended for this include using ivermectin on days 1, 2, 8, 9, and 15 plus permethrin 5 percent (total body) cream application for seven days and then twice a week until it appears to be gone. The patient may need to be isolated until the treatment is effective.

Key Takeaways

- There are oral, topical, and intravenous drugs used to manage fungal infections.
- There is a variety of drugs for malaria but they usually need to be combined for effectiveness.
- Chloroquine has the greatest problem with resistances with malaria.
- Antihelminthic drugs are given orally to kill or stun the worm.
- Pediculosis drugs can paralyze or suffocate the louse. There are oral forms of anti-lice treatment and topical treatment.

Quiz

1. Clotrimazole and betamethasone are used topically for the treatment of certain infections. Which one is not treated by this combination?
   a. Ringworm
   b. Thrush
   c. Athlete's foot
   d. Jock itch

Answer: b. The combination of clotrimazole and betamethasone can be used for any of the above fungal diseases but it is not used for thrush.

2. Monistat comes in several forms. What form is one that miconazole doesn't come in?
   a. Oral pill
   b. Vaginal suppository
   c. Topical ointment
   d. Topical cream

Answer: a. Miconazole is purely designed for topical use and isn't available as an oral medication.

3. Lamisil or terbinafine must be used orally in order to be effective in treating what fungal infection?
   a. Pityriasis versicolor
   b. Jock itch
   c. Ring worm
   d. Onychomycosis

Answer: d. It requires an oral medication of terbinafine in order to fight onychomycosis. The other disorders can be treated topically.

4. Which antifungal drug is reserved for serious and systemic fungal infections?
   a. Ketoconazole
   b. Fluconazole
   c. Itraconazole
   d. Amphotericin B

Answer: d. Amphotericin B is used for the treatment of severe fungal infections and is given intravenously.

5. What type of toxicity limits the use of amphotericin B in the management of fungal infections?
   a. Hepatotoxicity
   b. Renal toxicity
   c. Neural toxicity
   d. Cardiotoxicity

Answer: b. The biggest risk in toxicity of amphotericin B is that of renal toxicity, which is reduced by using liposomal amphotericin B.

6. Which cranial nerve is most affected by the excessive use of quinine products?
   a. Second
   b. Seventh
   c. Eighth
   d. Tenth

Answer: c. In the use of quinine for malaria, the main issue is toxicity to the eighth cranial nerve and hearing deficits.

7. What highly effective antimalarial drug comes from an ancient Chinese herb?
   a. Artemisinin
   b. Proguanil
   c. Mefloquine
   d. Quinine

Answer: a. Artemisinin comes from a Chinese herb that has been in use for thousands of years against febrile illnesses, including malaria.

8. What antibacterial drug is not among those also used for malaria?
   a. Doxycycline
   b. Tetracycline
   c. Metronidazole
   d. Clindamycin

Answer: c. Metronidazole is an antibiotic but it is not one of the more common drugs used for malaria.

9. What anti-parasitic drug is effective in second-stage African sleeping sickness and Chagas disease?
   a. Eflornithine
   b. Nifurtimox
   c. Suramin

d. Melarsoprol

Answer: b. Nifurtimox can be used in combination with other drugs to treat African sleeping sickness but is used as a solo agent in Chagas disease.

10. Which anti-lice treatment is specifically active because it causes suffocation of the louse?
    a. Benzyl alcohol
    b. Malathion
    c. Lindane
    d. Pyrethrin

Answer: a. Benzyl alcohol is known to kill lice through suffocation—something the other anti-lice drugs do not do.

Chapter 9: Sepsis

Sepsis is commonly associated with some type of bacteremia (which can be Gram-negative or Gram-positive sepsis) and the body's adverse reaction to the bloodborne organism. Sepsis is often accompanied by a systemic inflammatory response and multiple organ dysfunction. Many people who die of sepsis have death secondary to multiple organ failure stemming from the overwhelming inflammatory response to the infection.

Bacterial Sepsis

The diagnosis of bacterial sepsis depends on the presence of bacteria and the coexistence of a systemic inflammatory response. There is a subset called severe sepsis, which also involves organ dysfunction or organ failure. There is a subset of this called "septic shock" where there is a collection of cellular, circulatory, and metabolic problems leading to hypotension. Hypotension is regarded as having a blood pressure level that requires vasopressors with a serum lactate level of greater than 2 mmol per liter after fluid resuscitation.

Figure 23 shows the overall pattern of sepsis:

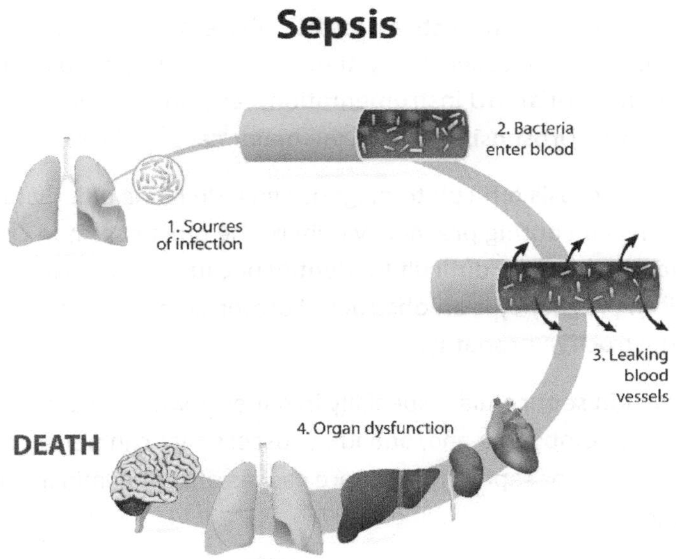

Figure 23

Things that can lead to sepsis include pneumonia, bowel perforation or ruptured intraabdominal/pelvic structure, pyelonephritis, renal abscess (within or around the kidney), acute prostatitis, or prostatic abscess. Any of these can lead to bacteremia, which initiates the process of sepsis.

The phenomenon of sepsis is complicated and stems from cytokine release caused by bacteria in the bloodstream. All of the clinically-observable findings in sepsis come from the cytokine release, causing decreased blood pressure, decreased organ perfusion, and impairment of liver function, kidney function, and lung function. Without the excessive cytokine release, sepsis would be much less severe.

Signs and Symptoms of Sepsis

The patient's history and physical examination might suggest the source of the infection and the presence of sepsis. The patient will often have a fever (plus or minus shaking chills), impairment of mental status (from hypoperfusion or high fever), tachypnea (leading to respiratory alkalosis), and cold or hot skin (depending on perfusion status).

An infected IV line can lead to bacteremia. Infections rarely occur from arterial or peripheral venous lines but may occur with long-term central lines. There may be evidence of a local central line site infection with redness and warmth of the site. Actual evidence of a local central line infection is present only 50 percent of the time.

A GI or GU source is suggested by having a known abdominal or genitourinary infection that has likely become bloodborne. The patient may have abdominal pain with the location of the pain indicating the possible source. Diffuse pain is from peritonitis or pancreatitis. Right upper quadrant abdominal pain suggests the gallbladder; right lower abdominal pain suggests Crohn's disease or appendicitis; left lower quadrant abdominal pain suggests diverticulitis.

Tenderness on rectal exam in males suggests a prostatic abscess. GU findings include known pyelonephritis, abnormalities of the collective system, stone disease, or costovertebral angle tenderness (suggestive of acute pyelonephritis). GU instrumentation, renal insufficiency, and urinary tract obstruction can lead to sepsis. Urosepsis is one of the major causes of Gram-negative septicemia.

Things that make abdominal sepsis difficult to diagnose include being elderly (in which peritonitis may not have classic symptoms) and during pregnancy (where the most common cause of sepsis is the urinary tract but, if abdominal, will be difficult to identify because of the rising uterus). The most common cause of sepsis in pregnancy is an obstructed ureter with urosepsis. The uterus will block the ureter and will lead to obstructive uropathy.

Pneumonia itself can result in septicemia, especially in patients with the actual or functional loss of the spleen. Infection can lead to empyema and/or a lung abscess that can persist and lead to bacterial septicemia and resultant sepsis or septic shock. Rare causes of septicemia include valvular abscesses and acute bacterial endocarditis.

Diagnosis of Sepsis

Testing that can help diagnose sepsis include a CBC (which can show an elevated WBC or low WBC count, low hemoglobin, or thrombocytopenia). Bacterial cultures of the blood can identify the bacterial organism responsible. If the IV site is suspected, the tip of the catheter should be cultured. Urinalysis and culture may help in the diagnosis. Gram staining of the buffy coat may reveal organism in the smear. This is the fastest way to get the diagnosis of a causative organism. A nasal culture is necessary for ruling out (or in) methicillin-resistant Staphylococcus aureus (MRSA). A positive MRSA culture of the nose may increase the suspicion of MRSA sepsis but does not necessarily correlate well with the positivity of the blood.

In cases of suspected urosepsis, the urine should be evaluated with a urinalysis, microscopy, Gram stain of the urine, and a urine culture. If urosepsis is the cause, the Gram-stain of the urine will be the fastest way to make a diagnosis.

Imaging may include a chest x-ray in order to look for a pulmonary cause of the infection, an abdominal ultrasound for biliary tract disease (including obstruction), and an abdominal CT or MRI (to look for renal or extrarenal causes of infection). The ultrasound is a good diagnostic tool for biliary tract disease but is not effective in detecting other causes of sepsis so the CT or MRI would be necessary.

Invasive procedures that may help include paracentesis (in cases of ascites), thoracentesis (with pleural effusions), and Swan-Ganz catherization (which is not for diagnosis but for following the fluid status). Aspiration of an abscess or lumbar puncture may need to be performed.

If the patient is not likely to have sepsis but in cardiogenic shock, an ECG should be obtained as well as cardiac enzyme levels. There are uncommon conditions when the patient may be suffering from an asymptomatic, "silent" myocardial infarction and will have shock in the absence of septicemia that needs to be ruled out in the differential diagnosis. Patients who are elderly, diabetic, uremic, or alcoholic will have a greater than average chance of having an MI as the cause of shock that isn't related to an infectious process.

There is a blood test that may be helpful in diagnosing bacteremia (if available). This is the procalcitonin (PCT) level. This can be accurate in determining the presence of septicemia about 94-99 percent of the time. Unfortunately, the PCT level is expensive and not available in many places. It may or may not be worth the cost of performing the test in terms of sparing unnecessary antibiotic use or altering the mortality levels of the patient.

Treatment of Sepsis

The goal of treating patients with sepsis is to treat aggressively with antibiotics based on the culture or the suspected location of the infection. Septic patients are remarkably ill, requiring ICU admission in many cases. The first goal is to find the offending organ or site of the original infection. Antibiotics administration should not be held for a positive culture, thus broad-spectrum antibiotics should be first-line therapy. Besides antibiotics, supportive therapy should be offered, including cardiovascular and respiratory support.

Surgical intervention should be considered in intraabdominal sepsis or pelvic sepsis. Surgery may be essential in treating the problem, particularly in cases of peritoneal abscesses. Inadequate drainage of abscesses in the chest, pelvis, or abdomen can result in failure to resolve the sepsis, despite adequate antibiotics and supportive measures.

The initial antibiotic choice depends on the presumed source of the infection. It must be able to cover for all of the possible pathogens before the culture returns. The most important part of the antibiotics isn't the choice of antibiotics, rather how soon antibiotics are administered. Regardless of the cause, the patient should be treated for about two weeks (after the cause has been identified and the surgical interventions have taken place). The only time antibiotics are recommended for longer than three weeks is with liver abscesses.

IV-line infections are usually caused by Staphylococcus aureus (methicillin-sensitive or methicillin-resistant) so this organism should be covered. The treatment of choice is meropenem or cefepime plus coverage for MRSA (which would include vancomycin, daptomycin, or linezolid). If the organism is not MRSA, vancomycin should be avoided and a more narrow-spectrum antibiotic is recommended. The reason for this is that it can encourage the growth of vancomycin-resistant enterococcus (Enterococcus faecium). Vancomycin should be used if there is central line infection and the line cannot be removed.

If the source of the infection is possibly or likely to be biliary tract in nature, the pathogens that must be covered for include Enterococcus faecalis, Klebsiella, and Escherichia coli. Anaerobes are necessary only in people who are either diabetic or are seen to have emphysematous cholecystitis (which would implicate Clostridium perfringens). When anaerobic coverage is not required, appropriate coverage may include imipenem, piperacillin-tazobactam, ampicillin-sulbactam, or meropenem.

Lower abdominal and pelvic infections include Enterococcus, Gram-negative bacilli, and Bacillus fragilis. Enterococci do not require coverage, however, the others do. The monotherapy for these include any of the following include imipenem, piperacillin-tazobactam, meropenem, tigecycline, and ampicillin-sulbactam. Dual therapy for these types of infections include either metronidazole or clindamycin plus an aminoglycoside, levofloxacin, or aztreonam.

If the patient is believed to have urosepsis, the organisms requiring coverage include Enterococcus faecalis, Enterococcus faecium, and Escherichia coli. Rare causes include Serratia, Enterobacter, and Pseudomonas aeruginosa (in instrumentation-caused infections). Treatment should start with a third- or fourth-generation cephalosporin, an aminoglycoside, levofloxacin, or aztreonam. If Enterococcus faecalis is the organism suspected or proven, the choice is vancomycin or ampicillin. If vancomycin-resistant Enterococcus faecium is suspected, then daptomycin or linezolid should be considered.

Staphylococcus aureus is the primary agent in acute bacterial endocarditis and in foreign bodies/devices. Nafcillin is the first-line agent, as well as any cephalosporin, linezolid, daptomycin, and carbapenem. Meningococcus or pneumococcus is treated with penicillin G or a beta-lactam. If the patient is believed to be septic from meningitis, the antibiotic must be able to cross the blood-brain barrier.

If there is no obvious cause for the sepsis, the sources to be suspected are the GU tract, the distal GI tract, and the pelvis. The main pathogens to be considered include coliforms (Gram-negative bacilli) and Bacillus fragilis. If urosepsis or biliary tract sepsis are suspected, Enterococcus should be covered for.

Prognosis of Sepsis

Sepsis is a common cause of morbidity and mortality with the outcome depending on the host defenses and the underlying health status of the patient. Early and appropriate treatment with the right antibiotic choice, along with surgical intervention (if necessary) will improve the outcome. Relief of obstruction of the urinary tract or biliary tract is needed to maximize outcome. The worst prognosis stems from patients with pelvic or intraabdominal abscesses from organ perforation. The underlying health of the patient is the primary determinant of patient survival.

Key Takeaways

- Sepsis stems from bacteremia and the body's systemic inflammatory response to the organism.
- The major causes of sepsis are from GI, biliary tract, GU, and lung sources. Less common causes are CNS-related or related to endocarditis.
- The main resistances to consider in sepsis are MRSA and VRE (vancomycin-resistant enterococcus faecium).
- The main goal of sepsis is to start an appropriate antibiotic as soon as possible.

Quiz

1. What is not necessarily present in cases of severe sepsis?
   a. Bacteremia
   b. Systemic inflammatory response
   c. Organ dysfunction
   d. Hypotension

Answer: d. There is not necessarily hypotension until it progresses to septic shock. The other things are present in cases of severe sepsis.

2. What type of infection is least likely to lead to sepsis?
   a. Intracranial infection
   b. Intraabdominal infection
   c. Pneumonia
   d. Urinary tract infection

Answer: a. Each of these can result in sepsis, with intracranial infections being the least likely to result in bacteremia and sepsis.

3. What type of acid-base abnormality is seen in acute sepsis cases?
   a. Metabolic alkalosis
   b. Respiratory alkalosis
   c. Metabolic acidosis
   d. Respiratory acidosis

Answer: b. The patient will have respiratory alkalosis because of tachypnea and because they are blowing off "acidic" CO_2, raising the pH of the blood.

4. What is the most common cause of septicemia and sepsis in patients who are pregnant?
   a. Ruptured uterus
   b. Acute appendicitis
   c. Obstructive uropathy
   d. Ovarian abscess

Answer: c. The most common cause of sepsis in pregnancy is obstructive uropathy from the ureter being obstructed by the expanded uterus.

5. What invasive procedure is least likely to be diagnostic in the identification of sepsis?
   a. Swan-Ganz catheter
   b. Paracentesis
   c. Thoracentesis
   d. Lumbar puncture

Answer: a. The Swan-Ganz catheter can be placed in order to manage the patient's fluid status but is not used as a way of diagnosing the cause of sepsis.

6. What is the fastest diagnostic test for the causative organism in acute sepsis?
   a. Blood culture
   b. Buffy coat staining
   c. Urinalysis
   d. Nasal mucosa culture

Answer: b. The quickest way to determine a causative organism in acute sepsis is the buffy coat staining, which will show the organism with just a Gram-stain of the blood.

7. What is the most common organism to be covered for in cases of suspected IV-line septicemia?
   a. Staphylococcus aureus
   b. Streptococcus pyogenes
   c. Streptococcus pneumoniae
   d. Haemophilus influenzae

Answer: a. Staphylococcus aureus and, in some cases, MRSA, should be covered for in cases of IV-line septicemia.

8. Which antibiotic choice is not considered most likely to be necessary for suspected MRSA coverage?
   a. Vancomycin
   b. Ciprofloxacin
   c. Daptomycin
   d. Linezolid

Answer: b. Each of these are proper choices for MRSA coverage except for ciprofloxacin, which doesn't cover MRSA.

9. The patient is suspected to have biliary tract sepsis. What organism does not have to be covered for in such cases?
   a. Escherichia coli
   b. Klebsiella
   c. Staphylococcus aureus
   d. Enterococcus faecalis

Answer: c. The organisms suspected in biliary tract disease and secondary sepsis are any of the above choices except for Staphylococcus aureus.

10. Which cause of sepsis carries the worst prognosis?
    a. Bowel perforation
    b. Meningitis
    c. Bacterial endocarditis
    d. Prostatic abscess

Answer: a. The worst prognosis in sepsis stems from a bowel perforation, which often leads to intraabdominal or intrapelvic abscesses.

Chapter 10: HIV Disease

HIV disease is caused by the human immunodeficiency virus, which is a type of retrovirus. The disease is transferred directly from one human to another through the exchange of blood or bodily fluids. The disease is not curable; however, there are several drug regimens for HIV infections that will slow the progression of the disease.

HIV Virus

The HIV virus or human immunodeficiency virus is a type of retrovirus of the subgroup lentivirus. It causes HIV disease that leads to acquired immunodeficiency syndrome or AIDS, which progressively results in a failure of the immune system. The end result is the development of several types of life-threatening opportunistic infections and certain unusual cancers. The average lifespan without treatment is 10 years (although it depends on the subtype).

Figure 24 shows an HIV virus attacking a human cell:

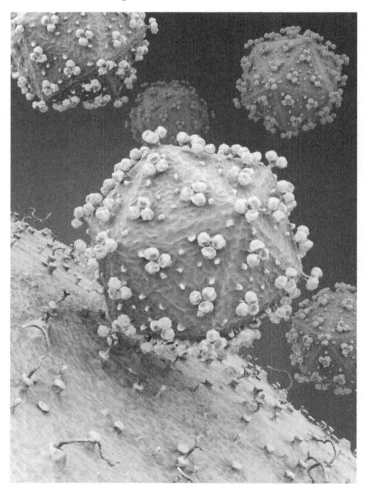

Figure 24

The disease is passed through the exchange of blood or body fluids, including semen, vaginal fluids, and pre-ejaculate. It can also be passed to an infant in utero or through breast milk. This means that HIV can be passed via the placenta (in utero) or via the vaginal secretions at the time of birth, with free viral particles and viruses inside immune cells able to pass along the disease.

The main cells infected in HIV disease include CD4+ cells (helper cells), dendritic cells, and macrophages (affecting the innate and adaptive immune systems). The end result is a decrease in helper cells, which get killed both as infected and uninfected cells. It is the CD8+ cell type that gets rid of the helper cells, which reach critically low levels.

There are two types of HIV viruses, HIV-1 and HIV-2. HIV-1 is highly virulent and infective, with global prevalence and a presumed origin in the common chimpanzee. HIV-2 is believed to have come from the Sooty mangabey. It is only seen in West Africa and has a lower virulence rate when compared to HIV-1.

The main characteristics of the Lentivirus genus (of which HIV belongs) is a long-duration of illness with a long incubation period. These are single-stranded, positive-sense RNA viruses. After it enters the cell, the RNA genome turns into a double-stranded DNA genome by an enzyme encoded by the virus called reverse transcriptase. The nucleic acid chain then gets transferred into the host nucleus by the virally-encoded integrase enzyme. The virus then becomes latent for up to ten years without causing symptoms.

HIV Is a spherical virus about sixty times smaller than an erythrocyte, consisting of two copies of its single-stranded RNA genome. There are nine genes in the capsid, which is made from the p24 viral protein. The main enzymes encoded by the viral genes are reverse transcriptase, proteases, integrase, and ribonuclease. There is a matrix made of the p17 protein that stabilizes the viral particle around the capsid. The viral envelope surrounds everything and is made from the lipid bilayer of the human host that the virus particle budded off from. A few copies of an envelope protein come from the virion called glycoprotein (gp) 120, as well as a stem made of gp41 molecules that keep the virus anchored to the envelope. The env gene in the virus encodes for the protein necessary to attach the virus to the infected cells.

The nine genes (pol, gag, tat, env, nef, vpu, vpr, and nef) encode for a total of 19 proteins. Just three of these genes (pol, gag, and env encode for structural viral proteins). The env gene encodes for the gp160 protein, that divides by means of a protease to make gp120 and gp41. The rest of the genes are considered regulatory.

The term known as viral tropism refers to the cell types that the viral particle infects. HIV-1 gains access to the cells it infects by an interaction between the gp120 (envelope glycoprotein) with the CD4+ cell membrane. There are only certain strains of the virus, called macrophage-tropic (M-tropic) strains of the HIV virus, that can gain entry into the macrophage via the CCR5 chemokine receptor. It is the macrophages and the dendritic (microglial cells) that get infected by the HIV virus in the CNS of the host. The patient will also have adenoid and tonsil infection with HIV, which produce cells that make large amounts of virus (from multinucleated giant cells in these tissues).

The replication cycle starts with an interaction between p120 and the CD4+ cell. This causes a gp120 glycoprotein conformational change that result in its interaction with the CCR5 receptor. The tips of the gp41 glycoprotein are inserted into the cell membrane. This causes the gp41 protein to fold in, forming coils. The virus is then pulled into the cell, with the membranes fusing. The HIV capsid enters the host cell.

After the HIV has entered the host cell, the RNA molecules and the different enzymes are injected into the cells. Reverse transcriptase starts its activity, leading to the RNA turning into double-stranded DNA, which in turn gets integrated into the genome of the host. There are two modes of entry possible for dendritic-tropic cells (the CCR5 receptor and the DC-SIGN receptor and related C-type lectin receptors).

Reverse transcriptase activation is very error-prone and can cause drug resistance against the drugs that work against this enzyme. There is ribonuclease activity that degrades the viral RNA while the complementary DNA (cDNA) gets made. There is also DNA-dependent DNA polymerase that makes sense DNA from the antisense cDNA that is originally made from the viral reverse transcriptase enzyme. The two DNA molecules combine to form double-strength DNA, which enters the nucleus of the cell and makes use of integrase to become incorporated into the genome of the host cell.

There is viral recombination that produces the genetic variation contributing to the evolution of the HIV particle and its resistance to anti-retroviral therapy. It also contributes to the ability of the virus to overcome the immune defenses of the host.

HIV Is spread via two means. The first is cell-to-cell spread and the second is cell-free spread. In cell-free spread, the virus exits the infected cell and enters the bloodstream in order to infect another T cell. It can also be spread to other cells via cell-to-cell spread, in which there is a virological synapse between the two cells or in which there is an antigen-presenting cell that transfers the virus from one cell to another. Cell-to-cell transfer occurs easier than cell-free transfer. This type of transfer is more efficacious in places like lymphoid tissues where there are a lot of CD4+ cells clustered together.

The HIV particle is different from other viruses in that it is highly variable genetically. It is partly because it is rapidly replicated (at about 10^{10} virus particles per day), a high mutation rate, and lots of recombination happening with the reverse transcriptase cavity. This happens to a greater degree when a person has two different HIV strains (which combine to form a brand-new strain).

There are three subgroups of HIV-1 that have different envelope regions (M, N, and O). Group M is the most prevalent and has eight separate subtypes, known as clades. These are geographically unique. The most prevalent subtypes of the M group are A and D (found in Africa), B (found in Europe and North America), and C (found in Asia and Africa). Subtype C is the most common type of HIV, accounting for 47 percent of all types of HIV disease. The European and American strains account for only 5 percent of cases.

Most HIV-infected patients do not know they have the virus. Only about 1 percent of urban Africans have been tested. Because of this unawareness, all blood products and donor blood are screened for the virus. The first test done is the ELISA (enzyme-linked immunosorbent assay), which is designed to detect the HIV-1 antibody. Non-reactive ELISA-tested blood is considered HIV-negative blood. A positive test is followed by repeated testing of the blood in duplicate with an ELISA test. The three possible follow-up tests include the IFA (immunofluorescence assay), Western Blot assay, or polymerase chain reaction. The IFA test is the least-common test for HIV. HIV-positivity is declared only if the confirmatory tests are positive. Patients with indeterminant Western blot tests should be retested in a month. Viral nucleic acid (RNA) testing is not commonly available but can help diagnose HIV disease.

The ELISA test is extremely sensitive and specific, leading to an accurate result more than 99 percent of the time. This leads to a false-positive test (in two-step testing) of about 1 out of 250,000 cases. The exposed patient is tested immediately, at six weeks post-exposure, at three months post-exposure, and at six months post-exposure. The immunoassay done must be for both HIV-1 and HIV-2 antibodies, as well as for the p24 antigen. A negative test means the patient is not infected, while any positive test needs further evaluation. The latest recommendations involve testing for the p24 antigen first; a negative test rules out an active infection.

HIV/AIDS

HIV/AIDS is a spectrum of diseases caused by the host's infection with the HIV particle. The patient may initially have no symptoms or may have an influenza-like disease. This is followed by a long period of time with no symptoms. The immune system gradually fails and both opportunistic infections and rare tumors develop. The late stages of the disease involve AIDS, in which the immune system is highly impaired and the CD4+ count is less than 200 cells per microliter.

The prevalence of HIV in people is about 37 million throughout the world with about 1 million deaths per year. Most of infected people live in sub-Saharan Africa with about 39 million deaths occurring in the world since the virus was first identified. This is considered a pandemic disease, having first been identified as a disease in 1981. The cause of the disease was identified several years later.

There are three primary stages of HIV infection: acute disease, clinical latency disease, and AIDS. Acute HIV disease is also called acute retroviral syndrome. It occurs 2-4 weeks after exposure as a flu-like or mono-like illness that does not occur in everyone. About 40-90 percent of infected patients will have clinical disease that includes enlargement of the lymph nodes, fever, rash, headache, and sore throat. There may be a rash in up to half of all cases, which is maculopapular and on the trunk. Opportunistic infections can happen during this phase. GI symptoms can occur, along with Guillain-Barre syndrome or other neurological symptoms. The symptoms tend to last about 1-2 weeks and are rarely identified as being HIV disease.

The longest stage of the disease is called the clinical latency stage, also referred to as asymptomatic HIV or chronic HIV. This stage lasts from 3-20 years without treatment (about 8 years on average). The disease is largely asymptomatic except for GI problems, myalgias, weight loss, and fevers near the end of the stage. About half to 70 percent of patients will have generalized lymphadenopathy involving more than one area over three to six months.

While most patients with latent disease have small viral loads, about five percent will have high levels of T helper cells even without antiretroviral therapy. These are known as HIV controllers or "long-term nonprogressors". About one in 300 infected people will have very low viral loads, called elite suppressors or elite controllers.

AIDS is defined as having CD4+ counts of less than 200 cells per microliter or specific diseases linked to an HIV infection that wouldn't be there in the absence of HIV disease. About half of people will have AIDS by the tenth year after infection. The most common things that trigger the diagnosis of AIDS include esophageal candidiasis, HIV-associated cachexia (20 percent), and pneumocystis pneumonia (40 percent). Recurrent upper respiratory infections can also indicate AIDS.

There are a variety of infectious diseases that can be linked to AIDS, including meningitis, encephalitis, retinitis, pneumocystis pneumonia, tuberculosis, rare infection-related cancers, candida esophagitis, and chronic diarrhea. Infections caused by bacterial organisms, viral particles, fungi, and parasites can happen, affecting just about every organ system.

Viral-related cancers include cervical cancer, Burkitt's lymphoma, Kaposi's sarcoma, and primary central nervous system lymphoma, with the most common cancer being Kaposi's sarcoma (occurring in up to 20 percent of patients with AIDS). Lymphoma causes 16 percent of AIDS deaths and identifies the disease in 3-4 percent of AIDS cases. Both Kaposi's sarcoma and lymphoma are secondary to the human herpesvirus 8 infection. Cervical cancer is related to the HPV or human papillomavirus infection.

About 90 percent of patients will have AIDS-related diarrhea, while others will have weight loss, weakness, chills, lymphadenopathy, fevers, and night sweats. There is a variety of neurological and psychiatric symptoms as well as opportunistic infections that can lead to the death of the patient for reasons other than simple AIDS.

The transmission of HIV can be through several different methods. About 90 percent of infected blood transfusions will lead to active disease. Twenty-five percent of children will get the disease through childbirth. Drug use with needles will lead to infection about 0.67 percent of the time (per injection). A needle stick causes infection 0.3 percent of the time. Lesser causes of HIV include receptive anal intercourse, receptive vaginal intercourse, insertive vaginal intercourse, receptive oral intercourse, and insertive oral intercourse. No other way of getting HIV exists unless blood is involved (sputum, saliva, sweat, urine, tears, or vomit).

Sexual intercourse is the most common way of getting HIV disease, with the most common sex being between people of the opposite sex (especially in Africa). Two-thirds of new cases in the US happen among homosexual men. About 15 percent of gay and bisexual men in developed countries have a positive HIV test, while 28 percent of transgender women will have HIV positivity. The rate of transmission is higher in low-income countries versus high-income countries. Among prostitutes in low-income countries, the risk per act of female-to-male transmission is about 2.4 percent per act. Genital ulcers increase the risk of disease by five-fold. Sexual assault and rough sex will lead to an increased risk of HIV disease.

The second-most common method of HIV transmission is through the exchange of blood products or blood. This can happen with needle-stick injuries, IV drug use, or blood product transfusions. Theoretically, things like tattoos with unsterilized equipment can cause HIV disease. It is possible to get HIV from mucous membrane exposure to blood but this is less common than a needlestick. IV drug users account for 12 percent of all new cases of HIV disease with some areas of the world having at least 80 percent of IV drug users being infected with the virus.

While there is a high risk of transmission with an infected batch of blood, the risk is less than one in 500,000 blood transfusions because HIV testing is done on all blood products. In poorer countries where HIV is not tested for in all blood products, about 15 percent of all new cases come from an infected transfusion. It makes up about 5-10 percent of all cases in the world. Tissue and organ transplantation can also cause HIV disease, although these are screened beforehand.

Vertical transmission from mother to child can happen during the pregnancy, at the time of delivery, or via breastfeeding. This is the third most common way of getting HIV disease in the world. The risk without treatment is 20 percent at birth and 35 percent with breastfeeding. About 90 percent of HIV in children happen because of vertical transmission. The risk can be decreased by having a cesarean birth, taking antiretroviral medications in pregnancy and childbirth, and avoiding breastfeeding. If the mother does breastfeed, taking antiretroviral agents will decrease the disease transmission. Untreated women who breastfeed will pass the disease on about 17 percent of the time (while treatment decreases the risk to 1-2 percent per year).

HIV Drugs

The management of HIV/AIDS involves using several antiretroviral drugs at the same time. The drugs will act on different aspects of the HIV life cycle. The treatment used on most people involves "HAART", which stands for highly active antiretroviral therapy. HAART will decrease the HIV viral load, preserving the immune system, and decrease the risk of opportunistic infections.

HAART is so successful that HIV has ceased to be fatal and has become more of a chronic disease, in which deaths from the disease are rare. There is no cure for HIV disease and the treatment only suppresses the illness. The risk of taking drugs is viral resistance, which is why multiple drugs are taken at the same time.

There are six different HIV drugs that are used in combination to treat chronic HIV disease and to prevent its transmission to other people. They address different areas of the life cycle of the microorganism. There are even fixed combination drugs used that will allow for fewer actual pills needing to be taken.

Entry inhibitors or "fusion inhibitors" block the entry of HIV-1 to the host cell. The two drugs available are maraviroc and enfuvirtide. Maraviroc binds to the CCR5 receptor that is found on CD4+ cells. CXCR4 is another receptor that the HIV particle can use as a form of resistance against these types of drugs. Enfuvirtide acts directly to prevent the fusion of the viral particle to the host CD4+ cell but must be injected.

NRTI or nucleoside/nucleotide reverse transcriptase inhibitors are analogues of nucleosides or nucleotides that block reverse transcription. They act as competitive substrate inhibitors to the reverse transcriptase enzyme so the process does not move forward. Examples of drugs of this class include tenofovir, emtricitabine, lamivudine, abacavir, and zidovudine.

Non-nucleoside reverse transcriptase inhibitors actually bind to the reverse transcriptase enzyme, acting as non-competitive inhibitors of the enzyme. There are first and second-generation NNRTIs. Among the first-generation drugs are efavirenz and nevirapine; among the second-generation drugs are rilpivirine and etravirine. They are only effective against HIV-1 disease.

Integrase inhibitors or "integrase nuclear strand transfer inhibitors" block the integrase enzyme. There are several of these drugs with raltegravir being the first FDA-approved drug on the market that does this. The compete with the magnesium ions at the binding site of the enzyme, effectively blocking its activity.

Protease inhibitors are able to block the protease enzyme needed to make mature viral particles after budding out of the host cell. The virus particles are defective and will not infect other cells. There are several of these drugs available, including ritonavir, amprenavir, atazanavir, darunavir, nelfinavir, indinavir, and lopinavir. The two first-line agents for HIV disease are darunavir and atazanavir. These drugs are ineffective alone as the resistance rate is high.

It has only been in the last decade that successful multiple drug strategies have been identified and used. Before that, many drug resistant strains were created and there were multiple-drug resistant mutations. Combination therapy can defend against this problem, reducing the chances of a mutation. HIV has a high mutation rate and a short life cycle so it can mutate to a superior organism quickly if not treated with different kinds of drugs.

The WHO guidelines for treating HIV disease with antiretroviral drugs includes using ART for all HIV-infected patients in order to decrease the risk of progression of the disease. While there are side effects associated with treatment, the benefits outweigh the risks. Combination therapy will decrease the rate of resistances and is available in drugs with fixed combination dosing.

Key Takeaways

- Human immunodeficiency virus is a type of retrovirus with single-stranded RNA.
- The disease is passed onto CD4+ cells, macrophages, and dendritic cells.
- HIV adversely affects the immune system and leads to cancers and opportunistic infections.
- The greatest transmission risk with HIV is with blood transfusions but this has been prevented by screening all blood products.

Quiz

1. Which part of the body is primarily affected by the HIV virus?
   a. Immune system
   b. Brain
   c. Liver
   d. Respiratory tract

Answer: a. All of the manifestations of HIV disease stem from a direct attack on the immune system.

2. What is the average lifespan of a patient with untreated HIV disease?
   a. 1 year
   b. 5 years
   c. 10 years
   d. 20 years

Answer: c. The average lifespan of a patient with untreated HIV disease is about 10 years (9-11 years, depending on the strain).

3. What is not likely to be a method of transmitting HIV?
   a. Placenta

b. Saliva

c. Vaginal secretions

d. Semen

Answer: b. HIV is passed through all of the above methods except for the saliva.

4. How many genes can be found in the HIV viral particle?
   a. 3
   b. 9
   c. 19
   d. 34

Answer: b. There are just nine genes found in the HIV viral particle that code for a variety of enzymes.

5. How many viral proteins are encoded for by the HIV genome?
   a. 3
   b. 9
   c. 19
   d. 34

Answer: c. The nine genes on the HIV virus encode for a total of 19 proteins.

6. Which glycoprotein is necessary for the attachment of the HIV viral envelope to the CD4+ cell?
   a. gp160
   b. gp41
   c. CCR5
   d. gp120

Answer: d. It is the gp120 protein that causes the HIV virus envelope to attach to the CD4+ cell.

7. What is the CD4+ count that is the marker below which the patient has AIDS versus just HIV disease?
   a. 100 cells per microliter
   b. 200 cells per microliter
   c. 800 cells per microliter
   d. 2000 cells per microliter

Answer: b. A CD4+ count of 200 cells per microliter or less is associated with the finding of AIDS versus simply having HIV disease.

8. What is the incubation period between the time of exposure to the time of acute HIV infection?
   a. 2-5 days
   b. 1-2 weeks
   c. 2-4 weeks
   d. 2-3 months

Answer: c. About 2-4 weeks after exposure, about 40-90 percent of patients will have an acute HIV infection that acts like influenza or infectious mononucleosis.

9. What infectious process or other process most heralds the presence of AIDS in HIV disease patients?
   a. Pneumocystis carinii
   b. Cachexia syndrome
   c. Esophageal candidiasis
   d. Kaposi's sarcoma

Answer: a. Pneumocystis carinii heralds AIDS in about 40 percent of cases, with the other symptom seen in a lesser percentage of cases.

10. What percentage of HIV cases in children stem from vertical transmission?
    a. 10 percent
    b. 30 percent
    c. 75 percent
    d. 90 percent

Answer: d. About 90 percent of cases of HIV in children stem directly from vertical transmission (from mother to child in utero, at birth, or through breastfeeding).

Chapter 11: Sexually Transmitted Infections

The main topic of this chapter is sexually transmitted infections or STIs. These include specific infectious diseases that are passed primarily from person to person through sexual activity and the exchange of bodily fluids. Many are bacterial diseases, which are curable through the use of antibiotics. Others are viral infections that cannot be cured but may be managed (in some cases) by using antiviral drugs. Several STIs are often contracted simultaneously in high risk patients, and need to be tested for and treated at the same time.

Gonorrhea

Gonorrhea is an STI caused by Neisseria gonorrheae. When symptomatic, it leads to symptoms of urethritis in men (with dysuria and penile discharge) and testicular pain. About 50 percent of men will have only urethral discharge. In women, it leads to dysfunctional uterine bleeding, pelvic pain, and vaginal discharge. About 50 percent of women will have symptoms. The main complication in women is pelvic inflammatory disease and the main complication in men is epididymitis. Both men and women may develop gonococcal arthritis or cardiac valvular infections.

Figure 25 shows the gonorrhea bacterium:

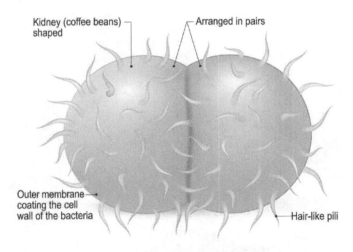

Neisseria gonorrhoeae

Kidney (coffee beans) shaped

Arranged in pairs

Outer membrane coating the cell wall of the bacteria

Hair-like pili

Figure 25

Gonorrhea can be passed via any type of sexual activity as well as to an infant from disease spread at the time of a vaginal birth. Infants can get an eye infection at birth called ophthalmia neonatorum. Because it is often asymptomatic, testing is recommended for all women under twenty-five years of age (annually) who are sexually active and after having a new sexual partner. All men who have sex with men should be similarly tested. Retesting is recommended for every person treated for gonorrhea after three months of treatment (as well as all sexual partners within the last two months).

The incidence per year of gonorrhea is about 0.8 percent of women and 0.6 percent of men. Most affected people are under the age of 25 years. Oral sex can lead to oral gonorrhea, with about 10 percent of patients developing a sore throat. The incubation period is about 2-14 days (average about 5 days). Rare cases can evolve into meningitis (especially in the immunosuppressed). Gonorrhea increases the risk of later having prostate cancer. There is no such thing as an immunity to the bacterium and reinfection is always possible.

The diagnosis of gonorrhea is done with a polymerase chain reaction of body fluids, which has replaced gram-staining and culture. Cultures are reserved for those who fail initial treatment. Testing for HIV disease, syphilis, and chlamydia should be done when the patient has a positive test for gonorrhea. The main treatment for gonorrhea is ceftriaxone (IM) along with doxycycline or azithromycin to cover for concomitant chlamydia. Treated patients should avoid sex for a week after final treatment for the infection.

Chlamydia

Chlamydia is an STI caused by Chlamydia trachomatis. Only 30-50 percent of women will have symptoms that can often take several weeks to develop. Symptoms in women include dysuria and vaginal discharge. Most women with chlamydia will get cervicitis and have mucopurulent discharge from the cervix. Half of these women will develop PID of the ovaries, fallopian tubes, and uterus, which can scar the pelvic organs. It can lead to pelvic pain that is not treatable and an increase in tubal pregnancies.

Figure 26 indicates the appearance of the Chlamydia organism microscopically:

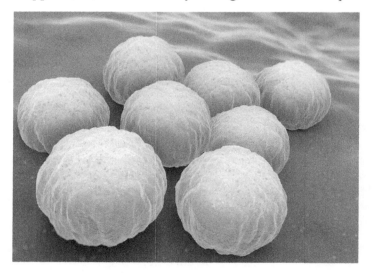

Figure 26

Men with chlamydia will have testicular swelling and dysuria. Men will have urethritis symptoms about fifty percent of the time, with urethral discharge, testicular pain, fever, or testicular swelling. The untreated infection can lead to epididymitis and infertility. It can lead to prostate inflammation but not to prostate cancer.

The main complication of chlamydia in women is pelvic inflammatory disease (PID). It is a major cause of infertility in women (who often for a while without treatment). In the developing countries, the infection can lead to trachoma (which is a roughening of the inner surface of the eyelids)—a major cause of blindness.

Any kind of sexual activities can lead to a chlamydia infection. It can be passed to the infant at the time of birth. Close personal contact with contaminated towels and flies will pass the disease in poor parts of the world. Screening is recommended at the first prenatal visit and annually in all sexually active women under the age of 25 years. Prevention is through using condoms.

The major treatment for chlamydia is azithromycin, doxycycline, erythromycin, levofloxacin or ofloxacin. Pregnant patients can be treated with azithromycin, amoxicillin, or erythromycin. Sexual partners also require treatment. There can be the resumption of sex when symptom-free and seven days after treatment. Repeat testing should occur after treatment, three months later.

Chlamydia is a common STD, affecting 4.2 percent of women and 2.7 percent of men. It is more common in women than men and is very rarely a fatal disease.

Syphilis

Syphilis is an STI caused by Treponema pallidum (a bacterium). There are four stages to the disease (primary, secondary, latent, and tertiary). It is spread through any kind of sexual activity or to a baby during pregnancy or childbirth, causing congenital syphilis. The testing for syphilis includes blood testing and looking for the bacterial species on dark field microscopy. All pregnant women are currently tested for the disease as a screening method.

Primary syphilis happens through direct sexual contact with a patient who has a lesion. A chancre (sign of primary syphilis) will occur 3-90 days after exposure. It is a single painless lesion about 40 percent of the time and multiple painless lesions another 40 percent of the time. The remainder of cases involve painful lesions that may not be genital. The cervix is the most common site of a lesion in 44 percent of women and is on the penis in 99 percent of heterosexual males. Gay men can have a chance in the rectal or anal area. Local lymphadenopathy is highly likely to occur.

Figure 27 shows a primary chancre seen in syphilis:

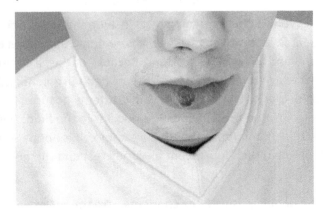

Figure 27

99

Secondary syphilis occurs about 4-10 weeks after the initial lesion is resolved. It involves a symmetrical, non-pruritic, maculopapular or pustular rash on the skin or mucous membranes, and lymphadenopathy. Warty lesions can also develop, which are infectious. Rarely the eyes and systemic symptoms can develop. Secondary syphilis can occur without a known previous case of primary syphilis.

Figure 28 shows the typical rash seen in secondary syphilis:

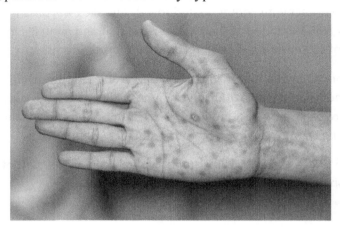

Figure 28

Latent syphilis is asymptomatic but there is a positive serological test for the disorder. It can occur months to years after resolving secondary syphilis. Patients with late onset latent disease are not as contagious as patients with early onset latent disease.

Tertiary syphilis can occur up to 45 years after the initial infection. There are three types: neurosyphilis, gummatous syphilis, and cardiovascular syphilis. About a third of untreated patients will have tertiary disease. The patient will have symptoms but will not be infectious. Gummas in tertiary disease are inflammatory lesions occurring anywhere on the body. Neurosyphilis involves a variety of neurological symptoms (including dementia, paresis, and seizures). Cardiovascular syphilis can affect the heart but primarily affects the aorta, leading to an aneurysm of the blood vessel.

Congenital syphilis happens in utero or at the time of birth. Only a third of babies will have symptoms. The symptoms happen over a couple of years and involves hepatosplenomegaly, fevers, rashes, pulmonary inflammation, and neurosyphilis symptoms.

There are different tests for syphilis. The screening tests include the RPR (rapid plasma reagin) and the VDRL (venereal disease research laboratory) tests, which are non-treponemal tests. False positives can happen in a variety of normal and abnormal situations. Because of this, a confirmatory test is done with a treponemal pallidum particle agglutination test (TPHA) or the fluorescent antibody absorption test (FTA-Abs). These tests become positive at about 2-5 weeks after exposure. Neurosyphilis is identified through CSF testing showing elevated protein and lymphocytes in the fluid. Dark field microscopy must be done on chancre fluid within 10 minutes of getting a sample. It is about 80 percent sensitive. Other chancre-related tests include the direct fluorescent antibody test and the nucleic acid amplification test, which is a PCR test.

Prevention of syphilis can be done by using latex condoms. Treatment of early infections is through the use of IM benzathine penicillin or, in PCN allergic patients, tetracycline or doxycycline can be used.

Patients with neurosyphilis can have IV penicillin or parenteral ceftriaxone. Treatment can be complicated by a Jarisch-Herxheimer reaction (fever, myalgias, and headache). Resistance to macrolides, rifampicin, and clindamycin is frequently the case. Sex should be withheld until the lesions have healed.

Late infections with syphilis require high doses of IV penicillin for at least ten days. Ceftriaxone is used for penicillin-allergic patients with neurosyphilis. Doxycycline or tetracycline can be used in late disease but for a longer period of time than in early disease. Treatment does not alter the adverse effects of the disease that have already occurred, such as can be seen with neurosyphilis.

Only about 45 million people have syphilis at any given point in time, with an annual incidence of 6 million infected patients. It is more lethal than most STDs, causing about 100,000 deaths per year. It had remarkably decreased in incidence when penicillin was developed but is seen in HIV patients, which has increased its incidence.

Human papillomavirus

The human papillomavirus infection is secondary to the human papillomavirus or HPV. Most infections have no symptoms and resolve on their own. Warts or precancerous lesions stem from different strains of the virus (of which there are more than 170 strains). Cancer risk is increased in the vulva, cervix, anus, mouth, penis, vagina, or throat. Almost all cases of cervical cancer are secondary to HPV infections (with most cases coming from an HPV16 or HPV18 strain). The other types of cancer are highly linked to HPV but not exclusively.

Figure 29 depicts the appearance of human papillomavirus:

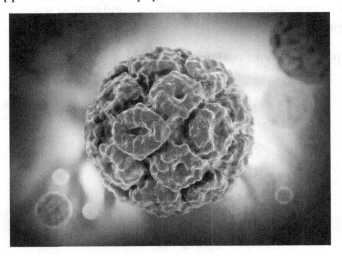

Figure 29

Venereal warts and laryngeal papillomatosis are both caused by HPV but are caused by different types than primarily cause genital cancers. HPV6 and HPV11 are typical causes of these warty diseases. The disease is spread through vaginal, anal, or oral sex but can be passed during pregnancy from the mother to the infant. HPV only affects humans and it is possible to have more than one type at the same time.

HPV is the most common type of STI in the world. Nearly everyone has had an infection at some point in their lives but most cases resolve spontaneously. About 1 percent of people have genital warts. Screening is done along with a Pap test. The only real treatment is freezing of the warts or other form of destruction (such as electrocautery). Precancerous lesions of the cervix can be treated with cryotherapy or conization of the cervix. There is no real effective cure for the disease unless it is eradicated physically.

There are three vaccines for HPV: Gardasil 9, Cervarix, and Gardasil. All will protect against HPV16 and HPV18. These are the two main cancer-causing viruses. Gardasil also covers for HPV6 and HPV11, which cause more than 90 percent of genital warts. Garadisil-9 covers for five additional types that lead to cervical cancer (31, 33, 45, 52, and 58). These are not helpful to people who've already been infected, which is why it is recommended for girls aged 11 to 12 years. Two shots, given six months apart, are recommended for children aged 11 to 12 years, with three shots given to older children. They are approved for both males and females but covered under most insurance plans for girls only in most countries.

Herpes Simplex

Herpes simplex involves any disease caused by the herpes simplex virus. Genital herpes results from an infection with HPV-1 or HPV-2. These infections can be asymptomatic or can lead to blisters and ulcerations. They break out and heal over two to four weeks, affecting the individual over and over again as there is no immunity built up to the outbreaks. Cycles of outbreaks can be months or years apart with the first infection being more symptomatic (leading sometimes to systemic symptoms). The episodes will decrease in frequency over time and will be less severe. It can, in uncommon cases, cause encephalitis, a finger infection (called a herpetic whitlow), and conjunctivitis. Babies can get it at the time of birth, resulting in neonatal herpes.

Figure 30 shows an individual with oral herpes simplex:

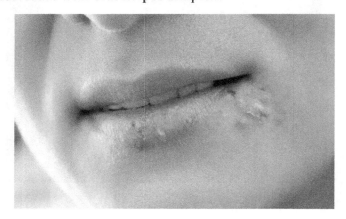

Figure 30

HSV-1 will mostly cause herpes of the mouth, while HSV-2 will mostly cause genital herpes, but the reverse can be the case. It is classified as an STI as it can be passed during sexual activity. The virus will settle in the sensory nerves after the first outbreak and will recur in cycles. The diagnosis can be made by obtaining a viral culture or by the finding of herpes DNA in blister fluid. Antibodies will be positive if there has been a past infection but won't detect new infections. Patients with known disease can take suppressive antiviral medications (acyclovir or valacyclovir) to prevent outbreaks. These drugs can be used also to decrease the severity of outbreaks.

HSV infections are the most common STI in the US, affecting about 60-95 percent of adults. Most people get HSV-1 as a child but get HSV-2 via a sexually transmitted disease. The prevalence of HSV-2 is about 16 percent, making it an extremely common STI. Most people do not know they've been infected but will be seropositive for the infection.

Key Takeaways

- Sexually transmitted infections can occur with just about any sexual activity between two people.
- Many STIs can affect a newborn in pregnancy or at the time of birth, causing neonatal disease.
- Bacterial infections causing STIs include gonorrhea, chlamydia, and syphilis.
- Viruses causing STIs include human papillomavirus and herpes simplex virus.
- There is a vaccine for HPV that can be given to boys and girls prior to becoming sexually active.

Quiz

1. What is the main complication of gonococcal disease seen in men with untreated disease?
   a. Cystitis
   b. Epididymitis
   c. Orchitis
   d. Pyelonephritis

Answer: b. A major complication of gonococcal disease seen in men is gonococcal epididymitis

2. What is a major complication of gonorrheal disease seen in women?
   a. Pelvic inflammatory disease
   b. Cervical cancer
   c. Ovarian abscesses
   d. Urethritis

Answer: a. A major complication of gonococcal/gonorrheal disease in women is pelvic inflammatory disease.

3. Which testing regimen is recommended for gonorrhea among gay and bisexual men?
   a. Test all men every 3-5 years while sexually active
   b. Test all men under 40 years of age at least once
   c. Test men under 25 years annually and with a new sexual partner
   d. No specific testing is recommended unless symptomatic

Answer: c. Men who have sex with men should be tested if under the age of 25 or who have a new sexual partner.

4. Which is not considered one of the three STIs are most commonly linked to one another that need to be tested for if one of the tests is positive?
   a. Gonorrhea
   b. Chlamydia
   c. HIV
   d. Syphilis

Answer: d. Syphilis is not a common STI and is not usually tested for if any of the other three become positive. The other three often coexist together.

5. Which STI is most linked to infertility in women?
   a. Gonorrhea
   b. Chlamydia
   c. Syphilis
   d. Human papillomavirus

Answer: b. The STI that is most commonly linked to infertility in women is chlamydia, which can lead to PID and scarring of the fallopian tubes.

6. Which antibiotic should not be used in pregnancy to treat chlamydia?
   a. Levofloxacin
   b. Erythromycin
   c. Amoxicillin
   d. Azithromycin

Answer: a. Each of these can be given in pregnancy for chlamydia except for levofloxacin.

7. Which stage of syphilis is mainly asymptomatic?
   a. Primary
   b. Secondary
   c. Latent
   d. Tertiary

Answer: c. Latent syphilis is rarely symptomatic but is identified by being serologically positive for the disease.

8. Which test for syphilis can be considered a screening test for the disease?
   a. Nucleic acid amplification test
   b. Rapid plasma reagin test
   c. Treponemal pallidum particle agglutination test
   d. Dark field microscopy

Answer: b. The RPR test or the rapid plasma reagin test is a good screening test for syphilis. It must be followed with a confirmatory test as there can be false positives.

9. What is the first-line therapy for patients with early or primary syphilis?
   a. Penicillin
   b. Ciprofloxacin
   c. Erythromycin

d. Tetracycline

Answer: a. A single dose of IM benzathine penicillin is recommended as a first-line therapy for early or primary syphilis.

10. Which strain of HPV Is not covered for with the Gardasil vaccine?
    a. 6
    b. 11
    c. 21
    d. 16

Answer: c. The four types of HPV covered for with the Gardasil vaccine include 6, 11, 16, and 18.

Chapter 12: Neglected Tropical Infections and Rare Infections

This chapter covers important yet neglected tropical infections and other rare infectious diseases. Diseases like dengue fever are highly linked to living or traveling to a tropical location. Other infectious processes are not necessarily seen in tropical areas but are more common in poor or rural parts of the world. Leprosy, rabies, typhus, and trachoma are rare infections that are not often encountered by the practitioner in developed countries but are important to be able to recognize and treat.

Dengue Fever

Dengue fever is caused by the dengue virus and passed through a mosquito-bite. The incubation period is three days to two weeks, with typical symptoms being headache, high fever, myalgias, arthralgias, vomiting, and a specific rash. People who recover tend to improve within a week; however, some can develop dengue hemorrhagic fever, associated with thrombocytopenia, bleeding, and loss of bodily fluids, leaning to hypotension and dengue shock syndrome.

Figure 31 shows the mosquito that transmits dengue fever:

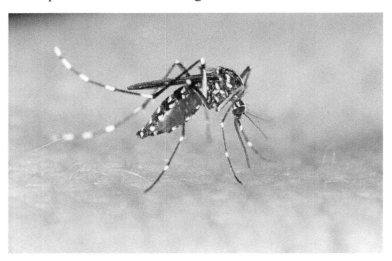

Figure 31

About 80 percent of infected patients are asymptomatic or have very mild febrile symptoms. Five percent have severe disease and the rare person develops shock. The average incubation time is 4-7 days. Children are at a higher risk of severe complications and GI symptoms. Fever is the most common symptom of all patients with the disease.

The disease follows a characteristic course with the sudden onset of headache and fever. There are three phases to the disease: febrile (with a 104 degree or more fever and headache lasting 2-7 days, petechiae, and measles-like rash), critical (with plasma leakage from blood vessels, decreased organ perfusion, and GI hemorrhage), and recovery (with resorption of fluid into the blood vessels lasting 2-3

106

days). People in recovery will have bradycardia and pruritis, along with a second maculopapular or vasculitic rash and peeling skin. Recovery isn't benign and can lead to cerebral edema, altered level of consciousness, and seizures.

There are several species of mosquito that can cause the viral infection. The genus is Aedes and the major organism is A. aegypti. There are five different types of dengue virus; however, immunity to one will lead to lifelong immunity to that virus and short-term immunity to the others. A repeat infection with another strain increases the complication rate. Dengue fever can be transmitted through organ donation or blood transfusions in endemic parts of the world. Vertical transmission is possible.

The diagnosis of the disease is primarily clinical although it can mimic other diseases. One test that helps diagnose the disease is the tourniquet test where a tourniquet is inflated, with petechiae of the arm noted after inflation. Labs will show thrombocytopenia, metabolic acidosis, and leukopenia. Elevated liver function tests are often seen. Leakage of plasma leads to hypoalbuminemia and a paradoxical rise in hematocrit from hemoconcentration. Ascites and pleural effusions are likely and can be seen on ultrasound. Signs of shock will be evident in severe disease.

The treatment of dengue fever is symptomatic and supportive. Patients can have oral rehydration therapy or IV therapy for 1-2 days until they begin to recover. The shock doesn't last very long and invasive procedures should be avoided because of bleeding complications. Acetaminophen can be given for fever (but NSAIDs and aspirin should be avoided). Blood transfusions are necessary for cases of a falling hematocrit. Platelet transfusions and fresh frozen plasma are not indicated. IV fluids are avoided in the recovery phase as there can be fluid overload. Furosemide may be necessary in the recovery phase.

There is a vaccine that is available in countries with a high risk of having the virus. Dengue hemorrhagic fever is one of the leading causes of hospitalization and death in children in many Southeast Asian countries, with Indonesia reporting the majority of dengue fever. The disease occurs only in humans and some non-human primates.

Other ways of preventing dengue fever is to use mosquito nets, wear protective clothing, and reduce standing water sources. Once contracting the disease, the treatment is supportive with oral or IV fluids. Hemorrhage and shock can be treated with blood transfusions and avoidance of NSAIDs. This is primarily a tropical disease but is actually a global health problem since World War II. It is a relatively common disease in 110 countries with up to 20,000 deaths per year.

The most severe dengue fever cases occur in babies and preschoolers, and is more severe in babies and kids who are well-nourished. Girls with a high body-mass index have a greater risk for the disease. The risk of severe disease happens if someone gets a DENV-1 disease, recovers, and then gets a DENV-2 or DENV-3 disease. Patients with asthma or diabetes can have worsened disease. People with certain gene mutations, such as HLA-B or G6PD deficiency have a greater risk for the disease.

Leprosy

Leprosy is also called Hansen's disease or HD. It is a long-lasting infection by one of two bacteria (Mycobacterium leprae or Mycobacterium lepromatosis). The infection is asymptomatic for 5-20 years with the development after that of granulomas of the eyes, skin, respiratory tract, and nerves. There can be paresthesias and anesthesia of certain parts of the body so wounds often go unnoticed. Other typical symptoms are decreased eyesight and weakness. Secondary infections cause tissue loss, resulting in loss of the tips of the fingers and toes, with the cartilage absorbed into the system.

The disease is spread via droplets between people and is much more common in poor parts of the world. Contacts of patients with leprosy are five to eight times more likely to develop leprosy than non-contacts. There are two main types of the disease (which is not very contagious). The types are differentiated from one another by the number of numb, hypopigmented skin lesions. The first is paucibacillary (with five or fewer lesions) and the second is multibacillary (with more than five lesions). The diagnosis is made by an acid-fast test of a skin biopsy or by detecting the organism's DNA in the tissue via a polymerase chain reaction.

The skin lesions may be isolate or multiple in nature and are generally hypopigmented. They may be nodular, papules, or macules. The classic finding suggestive of HD is that these are anesthetized areas of skin, which isn't the case with other skin rashes. Loss of sensation can be linked to muscle weakness. Skin smears are necessary for an accurate diagnosis.

Figure 32 shows what end-stage leprosy can look like:

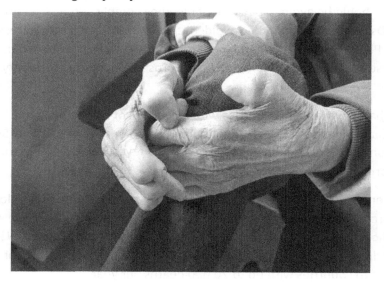

Figure 32

The microorganism responsible for the vast majority of infections is M. leprae—an aerobic, rod-shaped, acid-fast bacillus of the Mycobacterium genus. These are obligate intracellular pathogens that cannot be cultured outside of human tissue (making the diagnosis difficult). Molecular genetic testing is the only option for diagnosis. It can be grown in mice and other animals when injected with the bacteria. It is seen in non-human primates, red squirrels, and armadillos.

The treatment is curable with multidrug therapy. Paucibacillary disease is treated with rifampicin and dapsone for six months. Multibacillary disease is treated with clofazimine, dapsone, and rifampicin for twelve months. There are a select few of other antibiotics that can be used, all of which are given for free by the WHO. The number of cases has remarkably dropped to 230,000 new cases per year, which has decrease from 5.2 million cases seen in the 1980s. Only about 200 cases per year are seen in the US.

The best prevention is to detect the disease early and treat it, as the damage done is not usually reversible. Treating contacts will prevent the disease but WHO only pays for those patients who have symptoms. The BCG (Bacillus Calmette Guerin) vaccine offers about 26-41 percent effectiveness of protection against leprosy. A better vaccine is being studied for the disorder.

Rabies

Rabies is a viral illness that cause encephalitis in mammals, including humans. Typical symptoms include paresthesias at the site of exposure and fever. After this, there is excitement, violent movements, fear of water, confusion, paralysis, and coma (leading to certain death in 2-10 days if not treated). There is a 1-3-month incubation period (with a wide degree of variability). The virus needs to migrate from a peripheral nerve to the CNS to develop symptoms. Patients will be hydrophobic because of severe spasms of the pharynx and larynx with attempts to drink water.

There are two forms of the disease: paralytic and "furious". Hydrophobia is generally linked to furious rabies, which affects 80 percent of rabies-infected people. The remaining 20 percent of patients will have paralytic rabies that is marked by muscle weakness, loss of sensation, and paralysis. This type of rabies does not usually cause hydrophobia.

There are several viruses that can cause rabies, including types of lyssaviruses (such as the Australian bat lyssavirus and the "rabies virus"). It is spread when an infected animal species bites or scratches an uninfected person. Saliva touched to the mouth, nose, and eyes can also cause rabies. Dogs are the most common vectors, causing 99 percent of infections in places where they have dogs that are infected. In the US and the rest of the Americas, most infections are caused by bat bites (with only five percent coming from dogs). Rodents rarely cause the disease. Vaccination of dogs has led to a decrease in dogs as the vector in most parts of the world.

Any warm-blooded animal can get rabies and will have symptoms, including humans, birds, rodents, dogs, bats, and other mammals. It has also adapted to thrive in cold-blooded vertebrates so that most animals can be infected and will be vectors for human disease. Any wild animal can be a possible vector. The virus is present in the saliva and nerves of the infected animal with the bite of the animal being the most common source of the disease. The animal may be so affected that they bite without provocation. Human-to-human transmission is extremely uncommon but may occur with transplantation. Theoretical spread via sexual intercourse is possible.

The diagnosis of rabies is difficult, with the virus hiding in the nerves and in saliva. The fluorescent antibody test or FAT test is the WHO-recommended way of detecting the virus. Brain samples after death can easily make the diagnosis. Brain samples are the most sensitive way of getting the diagnosis, with the finding of Negri bodies (cerebral inclusion bodies) being 100 percent specific but only 80 percent sensitive.

Immunization of high risk people (who work with animals or bats) is the best preventative measure. Administering rabies immunoglobulin and the vaccine to people who've been exposed but don't have the symptoms is also effective. Wounds cleansed with povidone-iodine are at a decreased risk of passing on the disease. The disease caused death in about 17,000 patients throughout the world per year (mainly in Asia and Africa). Children are at higher risk for the disease. It is classified as a neglected tropical infectious disease.

There is an aggressive disease treatment called the Milwaukee protocol that will lead to a possible treatment in severely affected patients who don't have the vaccine or post-exposure prophylaxis. Using this protocol will result in a survival rate of 8 percent.

The CDC recommendation for treating the disease includes giving the vaccine in four doses over a two-week period of time and a single dose of human rabies immunoglobulin (HRIG). This is an expensive form of therapy and involves giving the HRIG as close to the bite as possible. HRIG that can't be given at the injection site should be given intramuscularly far from the site. The vaccine is given as soon as possible after a presumed exposure, repeating the dosing on days 3, 7, and 14. Patients who have already been vaccinated receive only two vaccinations at days 0 and 3. The vaccine is given in the deltoid muscle (and not the abdomen or gluteal muscles as recommended before).

Trachoma

Trachoma is defined as an infection with the bacteria Chlamydia trachomatis. It is specifically an eye infection, leading to a rough area of the inner aspect of the eyelid that rubs on the cornea, causing corneal breakdown and possibly blindness. It can lead to permanent blindness when untreated.

Figure 33 shows an eye infection from this organism:

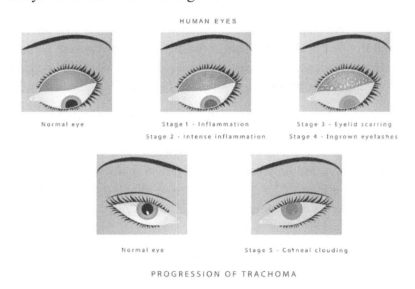

Figure 33

The incubation period of trachoma is 5-12 days, after which the patient has symptoms consistent with acute conjunctivitis. It usually takes multiple reinfections to cause the symptoms that lead to blindness. There are white bumps under the eyelids, usually in children. There may be follicles near the junction of

110

the sclera and cornea with a watery discharge. Some patients will get secondary infections, leading to purulent discharge.

Late stage disease causes structural abnormalities of the eyelid called "cicatricial trachoma". The eyelids invert so the eyelashes rub on the cornea, causing painful corneal abrasions and cornea opacities on healing. The follicles near the cornea will leave gaps in the tissue after healing (called Herbert's pits).

There are four stages to trachoma. In stage 1 (incipient trachoma), there is reddening of the palpebral conjunctiva. In stage 2 (established trachoma), there are follicles and papillae of the cornea and eyelids. In stage 3 (cicatricial trachoma), there is scar tissue of the palpebral conjunctiva and inverted eyelids. In stage 4 (healed trachoma), there is no active disease but the problems the cicatricial phase is still evident and blindness can be evident.

The chlamydia infection is spread via indirect and direct contact with an infected person's eyes or nose. Flies and clothing can harbor the infection that may then spread to the eyes, and the disease is more common with poor sanitation and crowded living conditions. This means that the best prevention is to improve sanitation and to treat those who have the infection as soon as symptoms develop. Whole groups of contacts can be treated with antibiotics to decrease the risk of the disease. Washing and proper hygiene is helpful, doesn't take the place of antibiotic therapy. Treatments include azithromycin orally as a single dose or topical tetracycline (in multiple doses)—with azithromycin being the treatment of choice. Surgery may be necessary to fix the eyelids.

The disease affects about 80 million people in the world, affecting up to 90 percent of children in poor parts of the world. The disease has cause total blindness in about 1.2 million people, primarily in Asia, Africa, Central America, and South America. If not treated, ulceration and scaring of the cornea lead to blindness. It can affect entire families.

Typhus

Typhus or typhus fever is actually a group of infectious diseases, such as murine typhus, scrub typhus, and epidemic typhus. The incubation period is one to two weeks with typical symptoms of headache, rash, and fever. This is a bacterial infection, caused by Rickettsia prowazekii. It is spread by fleas (Rickettsia typhi), chiggers (the cause of scrub typhus), and body lice (causing epidemic typhus from Rickettsia prowazekii). Queensland tick typhus is spread by a tick in Australia.

The most common form of the disease is epidemic typhus, leading to flu-like symptoms and high fever about one to two weeks after exposure. About 5-9 days later, a rash will spread from the trunk to the rest of the body. After this, the patient develops meningoencephalitis, leading to delirium and coma. Most untreated patients at this stage will die of the disease.

There is no vaccine for the bacterium with the best prevention being the reduction of exposure to the vector organisms. The main antibiotic used for the disease is doxycycline. The disease is seen in crowded areas where there is poverty and poor sanitation, particularly leading to epidemic typhus fever. Scrub typhus can be seen in parts of Australia, Japan, and Southeast Asia. Murine typhus is seen in tropical areas of the world, making this a neglected tropical disease. These are unrelated to typhoid fever, which is caused by Salmonella typhi.

Key Takeaways

- Many rare diseases are classified as neglected tropical diseases even if they aren't exclusively seen in tropical areas.
- Some rare diseases are viral, such as rabies and dengue fever.
- Diseases that are passed via bacterial infections include typhus, leprosy, and trachoma.
- Trachoma just affects the eyes and is a leading cause of blindness in the world.
- Vectors can cause several rare diseases, including mosquitos, vertebrates, chiggers, ticks, body lice, and fleas.

Quiz

1. What is the major mode of transmission of dengue fever?
   a. Fecal-oral
   b. Tick bite
   c. Tsetse fly bite
   d. Mosquito bite

Answer: d. Dengue fever is a mosquito-borne infection that is caused by a virus.

2. What is the most serious complication of dengue fever?
   a. Endocarditis
   b. Meningitis
   c. Shock
   d. Severe diarrhea

Answer: c. Some patients will develop loss of blood and fluids from infection and bleeding, resulting in dengue shock syndrome.

3. There are five types of dengue virus. What happens when the patient gets an infection from one of them?
   a. They have lifelong immunity to just the virus they contracted, and temporary immunity to the other types.
   b. They have lifetime immunity to all the strains of the virus.
   c. They have temporary immunity to all the virus strains.
   d. They have no immunity to any virus and can get the infection again.

Answer: a. The person who gets one type of the virus will get immunity to the virus strain that is lifelong but will have only temporary immunity to the rest of the strains.

4. What is the mode of transmission of leprosy?
   a. Droplet transmission
   b. Skin to skin contact
   c. Fecal oral route
   d. Insect vector

Answer: a. Droplet transmission through coughing or nasal secretions can pass on the disease.

5. The patient has paucibacillary leprosy. By definition, how many hypopigmented lesions do they have on their skin?
   a. One to two lesions
   b. Five or fewer lesions
   c. Fewer than twenty lesions
   d. More than five lesions

Answer: b. The patient with paucibacillary leprosy has, by definition, five or fewer hypopigmented lesions on the skin.

6. What is one way to diagnose a patient has having Hansen's disease?
   a. Positive serology for the organism
   b. Blood cultures for the organism
   c. Antigen testing of the skin tissue
   d. Acid-fast staining of affected skin

Answer: d. Acid-fast staining or PCR of the affected skin lesions will show the presence of the Mycobacterium organism.

7. What type of disease is rabies?
   a. Viral
   b. Bacterial
   c. Fungal
   d. Toxin-induced

Answer: a. Rabies involves a viral infection that travels to the CNS, resulting in seizures, coma, and death.

8. Which mode of transmission of rabies is not likely to result in developing the disease?
   a. Saliva touching the eyes
   b. Scratch by an infected animal
   c. Stool contact with infected animal
   d. Infected animal bite

Answer: c. Any type of contact with an infected animal, including saliva touching the eyes, nose, and mouth can result in developing rabies.

9. In developed countries of the Americas, what is the primary animal vector for rabies?
   a. Cat scratches
   b. Bat bites
   c. Rodents
   d. Dog bites

Answer: b. Bat bites are the main source of the virus in areas where dogs aren't known to be infected. In rare places, dogs can be the main vector.

10. Which antibiotic is most commonly used to treat typhus?

a. There is no antibiotic available
b. Amoxicillin
c. Doxycycline
d. Azithromycin

Answer: c. The treatment of choice for typhus is doxycycline.

Chapter 13: Nosocomial Infections and Opportunistic Infections

Opportunistic and nosocomial infections tend to be seen in patients who are hospitalized (nosocomial infections) or patients with a compromised immune system (opportunistic infections). The classically immunocompromised host is one with HIV disease; however, immunocompromised patients can have other conditions or may be taking drugs that affect their immune system. Nosocomial infections can affect patients with intact immune systems, but because they are hospitalized they are exposed to organisms that tend to cluster in these geographical areas.

MRSA

MRSA is also referred to as methicillin-resistant Staphylococcus aureus. This is a genetically unique Gram-positive bacterial organism that has evolved to be resistant to all penicillins, including methicillin. There is a general resistance to beta-lactam antibiotics, which include penicillins and cephalosporins. Strains that can be treated with these antibiotics are referred to as MSSA (methicillin-susceptible Staphylococcus aureus).

The organism is prevalent in prisons, hospitals, and nursing homes, where there are catheters, open wounds, and people who have poor immune systems. It is classified as a nosocomial infection. In rare cases, it can be community-acquired, associated with livestock or just in the community. Strains are also found to be resistant to clindamycin, oxacillin, erythromycin, teicoplanin, and vancomycin.

Staphylococcus aureus is part of the normal flora of the upper respiratory tract, skin, and gut. It can overgrow in these areas, leading to pathogenic disease. It can present on the skin as small maculopapular bumps that are erythematous, and associated with fever and sometimes systemic rash. The bumps turn into boils.

People at risk for the disease include people with catheters, drains, and prostheses, people who have poor immune systems, diabetics, IV drug users, people in crowded areas, the elderly, and users of quinolone antibiotics. Anyone staying in a hospital for a period of time are at risk for MRSA. College students in dorms are at risk. Some beaches in the US harbor the disease. People drinking unpasteurized milk and veterinarians are at risk. Hospital workers may harbor the disease. People with COPD or recent lung surgery can be at risk. However, about 22 percent of patients who contract MRSA will have none of these risk factors.

Hospital patients are at the greatest risk and can be treated with acceptable antibiotics. The disease can be spread from hospital workers to different secondary to poor handwashing techniques. Nursing home patients are immunosuppressed and may have catheters that harbor MRSA.

There is no quick way to diagnose MRSA so, if clinically suspected, coverage with antibiotic aggressively should begin before the cultures return. The fastest way to detect MRSA is a quantitative PCR test on suspected contaminated body parts. Rapid latex agglutination can also be performed that will detect the PBP2a protein on the MRSA organism that isn't found on methicillin-sensitive organisms.

Once diagnosed, or suspected, treatment of MRSA must be urgent as the disease can be fatal. The rout of administration of drugs to treat MRSA include IV or oral drugs. These organisms are resistant to beta-lactam drugs, including penicillins and cephalosporins. Community-acquired disease can also be resistant to clindamycin, tetracycline drugs, and sulfa drugs. The main eradication drug for MRSA is linezolid, although treatment protocols can vary depending on resistances. Linezolid will cure 87 percent of patients. Vancomycin is a second-line drug because there have been more resistances to MRSA (called VRSA). For MRSA pneumonia, the treatment of choice is clindamycin (if susceptible), vancomycin, or linezolid. Ceftaroline is a fifth-generation cephalosporin that can treat soft tissue infections secondary to MRSA or community-acquired pneumonia. Topical mupirocin is used to treat skin infections in children.

Pneumocystis Pneumonia

Pneumocystis pneumonia (PCP) is an opportunistic infection caused by a yeast-like organism (a fungus) called Pneumocystis jirovecii. It is not seen in immunocompetent hosts but is seen as a lung infection in patient who are immunosuppressed because of HIV/AIDS, chemotherapy patients, and those on immunosuppressive drugs.

Figure 34 shows the causative organism in PCP:

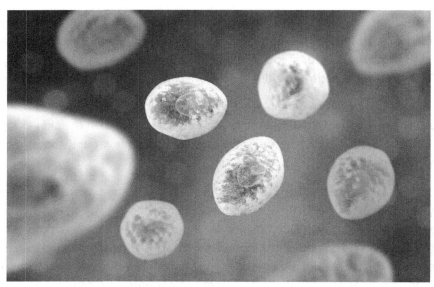

Figure 34

Typical symptoms include fever, dyspnea, non-productive cough, and night sweats. The sputum is too thick to be productive. There are rare cases of the organism spreading to the kidneys, liver, and spleen. A major complication of PCP is a pneumothorax. The risk increases in patients who have low CD4+ counts (below 200 cells per microliter). The patient with the infection will particularly have hypoxia and rising LDH levels. The alveoli become thickened, interfering with gas exchange and resulting in dyspnea.

There is a characteristic pattern on chest x-ray that can help diagnose the disease (with widespread pulmonary infiltrates) and low arterial oxygen levels. A Gallium 67 scan can detect the disease before the chest x-ray is positive. The organism can be found in the sputum or a bronchioalveolar wash. The organism can be found using a silver stain, toluidine blue stain, periodic-acid Schiff stain, or an immunofluorescence assay showing the cysts. A lung biopsy will show thickened alveolar septa with an eosinophilic infiltrate. PCR analysis is a newer diagnostic test of lung fluid.

Preventative measures include giving immunosuppressed patients atovaquone, pentamidine (inhalational methods), or trimethoprim/sulfamethoxazole. Steroids are given to decrease inflammation. Treatment should continue for 21 days with drugs like trimetrexate, pentamidine, atovaquone, dapsone, primaquine, and clindamycin (alone or in combination, depending on severity and resistances).

PCP is highly associated with AIDS and may be the first sign that the patient has an HIV infection. The first clue to the AIDS epidemic in the 1980s was the large increase in the use of the drug pentamidine. PCP was once a common cause of death in AIDS patients but the incidence has decreased dramatically because of the preventative measures taken using Bactrim or Septra (trimethoprim/sulfamethoxazole) in those patients with low CD4+ counts. In parts of the world without this preventative measure, the death rate from PCP is high.

Clostridium Difficile

Clostridium difficile, or C. diff, is an infection from the spore-forming bacterial species called Clostridium difficile. Symptoms include watery diarrhea, nausea, fever, and abdominal pain, causing about 20 percent of antibiotic-associated diarrhea. The major complications of the disease include toxic megacolon, GI perforation, pseudomembranous colitis, and septicemia.

The organism is spread through the fecal oral route with spores found in the feces that contaminate surfaces. Poor handwashing techniques will spread the infection in hospitals. Risk factors for the disease include being on antibiotics, being sick in a hospital, being of an older age, or using proton pump inhibitors. The stool can be tested via a toxin test, PCR test, or stool culture. Some patients will harbor the organism in the stool but will be asymptomatic.

Clostridium difficile is found normally in 2-5 percent of people. It produces several toxins that can affect the bowel, including enterotoxin (Clostridium difficile toxin A) and cytotoxin (Clostridium difficile toxin B). Both of these lead to colon inflammation and diarrhea. There is a third toxin that has been identified, called binary toxin, but it is unclear what effects it has on the patient.

The increased risk of the disease is most commonly used with clindamycin, cephalosporin, and fluoroquinolone usage. People around livestock where antibiotics are used are also at risk. Anyone in a hospital or nursing home is at an increased risk. As it is passed through the fecal-oral route, it is passed from one infected person to another through healthcare workers not washing their hands. Up to 50 percent of patients staying in a hospital longer than four weeks will get the infection. In the community, patients on histamine-2 blockers and proton pump inhibitors are at an increased risk for developing the disease.

Prevention of the disease involves judicious antibiotic use in patients, careful handwashing, and room cleaning after a patient is discharged from the hospital. About twenty percent of patients will have resolution of their disease with no treatment except for stopping the antibiotics in question. The rest can be treated with vancomycin, fidaxomicin, or metronidazole. Continued colonization is common, with recurrences in up to 25 percent of cases. Probiotics may help decrease the recurrence risk.

Cytomegalovirus

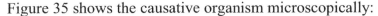

Cytomegalovirus or CMV can cause a wide range of infections, primarily a mononucleosis-type of disease but without a sore throat. Focal diseases (such as retinitis) can happen in immunocompromised hosts (like transplant patients, cancer patients, neonates, and HIV/AIDS patients).

Figure 35 shows the causative organism microscopically:

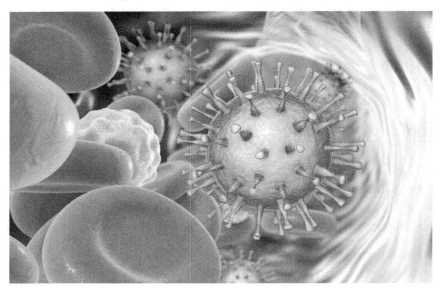

Figure 35

CMV is also referred to as human herpesvirus type 5 and is transmitted through transplanted organs, body fluids, blood, in utero, or at the time of a vaginal birth. About 60-90 percent of adults have had the infection, with lifelong immunity. Congenital disease can have no symptoms or can lead to miscarriage and postnatal death from liver damage and CNS involvement. A major finding is elevated liver function studies secondary to hepatic involvement and a proliferation of atypical lymphocytes in the bloodstream. The symptoms tend to last for 2-3 weeks. It is a major cause of infection and death in immunosuppressed patients, causing retinitis in up to 40 percent of affected patients. Still other sites of infection are the colon and esophagus.

Diagnosis of the disease can be done in several ways. PCR testing or antigen testing can identify the infection. A biopsy may show the virus and serology can identify CMV antibodies. Things like a Mono Spot will rule out EBV as a cause and hepatitis testing can rule out other causes of hepatitis. Lab testing for CMV is only necessary when trying to rule out other, treatable diseases.

In immunocompromised hosts, the disease is not always a new infection but will be a reinfection or reactivation of latent disease. The virus will be found in the urine, tissues, and other bodily fluids, which may or may not mean a symptomatic infection (and just represents shedding of the virus). Invasive disease can only be identified by tissue biopsy of infected tissues. Quantitative antigen or DNA testing of the blood can detect active disease as well. Only neonates can be diagnosed with a urine culture.

The treatment of choice for systemic and serious disease include ganciclovir, cidofovir, foscarnet, and valganciclovir. Retinitis is almost exclusively seen in AIDS patients and is treated systemically with any of the appropriate antiviral drugs. Prevention involves giving antiviral agents to high-risk patients, including those with HIV and transplant patients.

Kaposi's Sarcoma

Kaposi sarcoma or KS is caused by the human herpesvirus type 8. It is mainly seen in transplant patients and AIDS patients. The diagnosis is made by doing a biopsy of the lesion. It is a type of skin cancer that originates in endothelial cells infected with the herpesvirus type 8 virus; it is almost exclusively a disease of the immunosuppressed. The cancer looks like undifferentiated spindle-shaped smooth muscle or fibroblast cells.

Figure 36 depicts the viral particle microscopically:

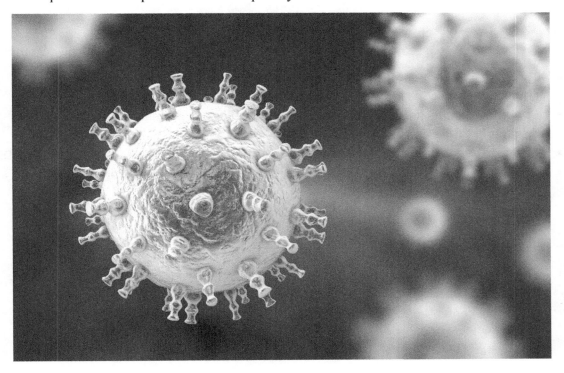

Figure 36

Classic Kaposi sarcoma in people who don't have immunosuppression involves being over 60 years, male, and of Eastern European, Jewish, or Italian descent. It is an indolent disease with a few lesions of the lower extremities, rare organ involvement, and a nonfatal outcome.

AIDS-related Kaposi sarcoma is the most common AIDS-linked cancer. It is much more aggressive than the classic form of the disease. There are multiple skin lesions affecting the face and trunk. There is frequent involvement of the mucosa, lymph nodes, and GI tract. It may be the first finding seen in AIDS patients.

Endemic Kaposi sarcoma occurs in Africa without an HIV infection. There is a classic form of the disease that is similar to classic KS, and a prepubertal form that affects children and involves the lymph nodes. Iatrogenic KS happens several years after a person has had an organ or tissue transplant and is on immunosuppressive drugs. Like AIDS-associated disease, it is more aggressive.

While this is primarily a skin cancer, it is necessary to evaluate the immunosuppressed patient for visceral involvement by doing a CT of the chest or abdomen. If there is no evidence of disease but symptoms of either pulmonary or GI disease, then an endoscopy or bronchoscopy is necessary.

The main treatment of Kaposi sarcoma is to do surgical excision, electrocautery, or cryotherapy to destroy the lesion. Imiquimod can also be used for superficial disease. Local radiation can destroy multiple lesions or lymph node-related disease. Antiretroviral therapy or interferon alpha can be used for HIV patients with systemic disease. Patients with iatrogenic KS can have a reduction in their immunosuppression to control the disease. Slowly-growing lesions do not have to be treated. Intralesional vinblastine can be effective.

Key Takeaways

- There are nosocomial infections associated with being hospitalized and often because of antibiotic use (such as MRSA and Clostridium difficile infections).
- Opportunistic infections and cancers stem from having a poor immune system (including diseases like CMV, Pneumocystis pneumonia, and Kaposi sarcoma).
- Often, an opportunistic infection is the first sign that an HIV patient has progressed to AIDS.
- Other immunosuppressed patients besides HIV diseased-patients include those on drugs after a transplant.

Quiz

1. What is the least likely geographic area to find MRSA?
   a. Prison
   b. Daycare center
   c. Nursing home
   d. Hospital

Answer: b. While MRSA can be found in the community, the least likely place to find MRSA is the daycare center. It is prevalent in the other areas listed.

2. In which place in the body would S. aureus least likely be resident as part of the microflora in the body?
   a. Skin
   b. GI tract
   c. Bladder

    d. Upper respiratory tract

Answer: c. The microflora of the skin, GI tract, and upper respiratory tract will naturally contain S. aureus, occasionally including MRSA.

3. What is the fastest and most effective way to detect MRSA?
    a. PCR test of infected fluid or nasal swab.
    b. Culture of the blood or body fluid
    c. Gram-stain of affected fluid
    d. Antibody testing of the blood for the MRSA bacteria

Answer: a. PCR testing can be done on infected body areas that will quantitate the presence of MRSA.

4. What is the main complication seen in patients with pneumocystis pneumonia?
    a. Pleural effusion
    b. Pneumothorax
    c. Lung abscess
    d. Spread to other organs

Answer: b. Pneumothorax is the major complication of pneumocystis pneumonia, which results in acute worsening in symptoms.

5. The patient is suspected of having pneumocystis pneumonia. A bronchoalveolar wash is obtained. What is not something that can be done with it to rapidly identify the organism?
    a. Silver staining of the wash
    b. Periodic acid Schiff staining of the wash
    c. Immunofluorescence assay
    d. Fungal culture of the wash

Answer: d. Each of these is a quick way of identifying pneumocystis except for a fungal culture, which is not a rapid detection test for the organism.

6. What is the main preventative drug used to manage the incidence of pneumocystis pneumonia in patients with AIDS and low CD4+ counts?
    a. Trimethoprim/sulfamethoxazole
    b. Doxycycline
    c. Clindamycin
    d. Pentamidine

Answer: a. The preventative measure of choice for PCP in immunosuppressed patients is trimethoprim/sulfamethoxazole or Bactrim.

7. What type of herpesvirus is cytomegalovirus?
    a. Type 3
    b. Type 5
    c. Type 8
    d. Type 10

Answer: b. Cytomegalovirus is also called human herpesvirus type 5.

8. Which organ is not a typical site where cytomegalovirus causes disease?
   a. CNS
   b. Liver
   c. Eyes
   d. Kidneys

Answer: d. The kidneys are the least likely place to find active disease, while the others are areas that are common places for a CMV infection.

9. What test can identify a patient who has had a CMV infection?
   a. Antibody testing
   b. PCR testing
   c. Tissue biopsy
   d. Antigen testing for CMV

Answer: a. Only antibody testing for CMV will indicate a past infection with CMV. Up to 90 percent of healthy adults will have had the infection at some point in their lives and will be considered "seroconverted".

10. What type of Kaposi sarcoma happens several years after having an organ or tissue transplant?
    a. Iatrogenic KS
    b. Classic KS
    c. Endemic KS
    d. AIDS-associated KS

Answer: a. Iatrogenic KS is a type of KS that stems from having had a tissue or organ transplant and usually occurs years after the transplant.

Summary

The topic of infectious disease is an important part of the study of internal medicine. It starts with the study of the host immune system. Many different types of organisms can overwhelm the host defense system to cause infectious diseases. Bacterial and viral diseases are extremely common infectious diseases, while protozoal diseases and parasitic diseases are less well-known. These disorders are primarily treated with antimicrobial medications. Infectious diseases that merit special attention were also discussed in this course, including HIV disease, sepsis, neglected tropical diseases, nosocomial infections, sexually-transmitted diseases, and opportunistic infections.

The human immune system represents the host defense system, which was the topic of chapter one in the course. There are two major components to the immune system, including the innate (nonspecific) immune system and the adaptive (specific) immune system. Each of these parts of the immune system have acellular and cellular components. This chapter provided a brief understanding of the innate and adaptive immune system and how they fight infectious diseases.

Bacterial infections commonly seen in humans was the subject of chapter two. There are infections that can arise spontaneously from a break in the protective barriers, such as the GI tract, respiratory tract, and skin. There are others that start as viral infections that turn into bacterial infections when the host is compromised by the initial infection. Bacteria are unicellular organisms further defined as Gram-positive, Gram-negative, and Acid-Fast bacteria, that can commonly infect humans. Different bacterial infections were also discussed in the chapter.

The subject of chapter three included common viral infections. For the most part, viral infections are more common than bacterial infections. While there are antiviral treatments some viral infections, many resolve spontaneously due to the patient's own immune system. Infections with viruses can be systemic or localized to a certain body area, such as the respiratory tract, liver, or gastrointestinal tract.

The topic of discussion was common fungal infections. Fungal diseases can range from minor to more severe diseases requiring aggressive therapy. Fungal organisms are similar to human cells so they tend to be more difficult to kill without causing significant side effects. Common fungal diseases such as Aspergillosis, Candidiasis, Histoplasmosis, Cryptococcosis and Coccidiomycosis were covered in this chapter.

In chapter five of the course, there was a comprehensive discussion of protozoal diseases. Protozoa are unicellular, eukaryotic, and non-photosynthetic organisms. Some protozoal infections are enteric in nature, leading to roughly the same symptoms from organism to organism. Other protozoal diseases, such as malaria, affect other body areas like the blood. Protozoal diseases can be seen in developed countries but more common in developing countries of the world.

In chapter six of the course, there was a discussion of common human-host parasitic diseases. While protozoa are considered parasitic, this chapter talked about some of the other parasitic diseases, including those caused by endoparasites (which cause internal disease) and those caused by ectoparasites (which cause external human disease). Parasites are known to cause a type of human disease called a parasitosis. Most parasites don't cause any disease, but other parasites have the potential to infect most living organisms.

In chapter seven, the topic was antimicrobial medications, known as antibiotics, and antiviral drugs. There are dozens of antibiotics that vary according to their mechanism of action on different bacterial organisms. Some antibiotics are bactericidal and kill bacteria outright, while others are bacteriostatic, and only stop the growth of bacteria, requiring an intact immune system to eliminate the bacterial infections. Drugs that act against viruses mainly attack an element of the life cycle of viruses, while there are a select few that act by enhancing the immune system's response to the viral organism.

Chapter eight covered the broad topic of antifungal medications, anti-protozoal medications, and anti-parasitic medications. The antifungal drugs can be topical, intravenous, or oral. Anti-protozoal drugs are generally oral drugs and vary greatly depending on the protozoal organism being treated. Anti-parasitic drugs can be taken orally for things like helminthiasis or used externally for ectoparasitic diseases, such as scabies and pediculosis infestations.

Sepsis was covered in chapter nine. Sepsis is a unique infection, involving some type of bacteremia (which can be Gram-negative or Gram-positive sepsis) and the body's adverse reaction to the bloodborne organism. Sepsis is often accompanied by a systemic inflammatory response and multiple organ dysfunction. Many people who die of sepsis have death secondary to multiple organ failure stemming from the overwhelming inflammatory response to the infection.

The focus of chapter was the spectrum of HIV/AIDS and the virus behind these diseases. HIV disease is caused by the human immunodeficiency virus, which is a type of retrovirus. The disease is transferred directly from one human to another by an exchange of blood or bodily fluids. The disease is not curable; however, there are several drug regimens for HIV infections that will slow the progression of the disease.

The main topic of chapter ten was sexually transmitted infections or STIs. These are infectious diseases that are passed from person to person through sexual activity and the exchange of bodily fluids. Many are bacterial diseases, which are curable through the use of antibiotics. Others are viral infections that cannot be cured but may be managed (in some cases) by using antiviral drugs. Several STIs are often contracted simultaneously in high risk patients, and need to be tested for and treated at the same time.

Chapter twelve covered some of the more important (yet neglected) tropical infections and other rare infectious diseases. Mosquito-borne diseases like dengue fever are highly linked to living or traveling to a tropical location. Other infectious processes are not necessarily seen in tropical areas but are more common in poor or rural parts of the world. Leprosy, rabies, typhus, and trachoma are rare infections that are not often seen by the practitioner in developed countries but important to recognize and have the ability to treat.

The focus of chapter thirteen discussed opportunistic and nosocomial infections. These are infections that commonly affect patients who are hospitalized (nosocomial infections) or patients with a compromised immune system (opportunistic infections). The classically immunocompromised host is one with HIV disease; however, immunocompromised patients can have other conditions or may be taking drugs that affect their immune system. Nosocomial infections can affect patients with intact immune systems who become ill because they are hospitalized and there are organisms that tend to cluster in these geographical areas.

Course Questions and Answers

1. Which cell type does not reside in the tissues as part of the innate immune system?
   a. Neutrophil
   b. Mast cell
   c. Kupffer cell
   d. Histiocyte

Answer: a. All of the cells listed commonly reside in the tissues as part of the innate immune system except for the neutrophils, which are floating in the bloodstream and recruited to the site of infection through the process of chemotaxis.

2. Which is not considered a localized symptom of inflammation?
   a. Tissue swelling
   b. Redness of the affected area
   c. Pain at the site of the infection
   d. Fever

Answer: d. Each of these is a localized symptom of inflammation except for fever, which is a generalized response to inflammation.

3. Where in the body are complement proteins generally produced?
   a. Leukocytes
   b. Hepatocytes
   c. Thymus
   d. Bone marrow

Answer: b. It is the hepatocytes that are responsible for making complement proteins.

4. Which type of cell in the immune system lives is in tissues and presents antigens to T cells as part of the adaptive immune system?
   a. Mast cell
   b. Eosinophil
   c. Dendritic cell
   d. Histiocyte

Answer: c. It is the dendritic cell that lives in the tissues and presents antigens to the T cell as part of the adaptive immune system.

5. Which are the main immune cells that attack tumor cells instead of pathogens?
   a. Histiocytes
   b. Natural killer cells
   c. Eosinophils
   d. Basophils

Answer: b. Natural killer cells are unable to kill pathogens but instead kill tumor cells or cells that are damaged in some way.

6. In phagocytosis, the oxygen-dependent portion of degradation depends on the creation of what molecule that is destructive to bacteria?
   a. NAPDH
   b. Hypochlorite
   c. Hydrogen peroxide
   d. Lysozyme

Answer: b. Hypochlorite is produced by the phagolysosome in an oxygen-dependent way and is destructive to the bacterium taken up by the organelle.

7. Which type of cell in the adaptive immune system functions to stimulate B cells to make antibodies?
   a. Cytotoxic T cell
   b. Antigen-presenting cell
   c. TH1 cell
   d. TH2 cell

Answer: d. A TH2 cell is a specialized T cell that activates B cells in order for the B cell to make antibodies.

8. Which type of cell in the adaptive immune system functions to kill pathogens directly, without using the cytokine system?
   a. Antigen-presenting cell
   b. Cytotoxic T cell
   c. TH1 cell
   d. T helper cell

Answer: b. A cytotoxic T cell functions to kill pathogens directly, without the use of the cytokine system. They are activated by the antigen-presenting cells and stimulated to kill pathogens.

9. Cell-mediated immunity functions does all of the following actions except?
   a. Killing virus-infected cells
   b. Killing intracellular bacteria
   c. Making antibodies against allergens
   d. Transplant rejection

Answer: c. Cell-mediated immunity does not make antibodies, which is part of the humoral immune system.

10. Which type of T cell is considered part of the innate immune system?
    a. Alpha beta cells
    b. Gamma delta cells
    c. CD4+ cells
    d. CD8+ cells

Answer: b. Of all of these cell types, only gamma delta cells are considered a part of the innate immune system.

11. What is another name for helper T cells?

a. CD4+ cells
b. CD8+ cells
c. Antigen-presenting cells
d. Effector cells

Answer: a. Helper T cells are also referred to as CD4+ cells because they express the CD4+ glycoprotein on their cell surface. They have different helper functions in the immune system and function in the cell-mediated immune system.

12. Which cells in the immune system function mainly to suppress the activity of cytotoxic T cells?
    a. CD4+ cells
    b. CD8+ cells
    c. Regulatory T cells
    d. Helper T cells

Answer: c. Regulatory T cells can suppress the action of cytotoxic T cells, which is important in the prevention of autoimmune diseases.

13. What is not considered a risk factor for cellulitis?
    a. Diabetes
    b. Lymphedema
    c. Obesity
    d. Renal failure

Answer: d. Each of these is a risk factor for cellulitis except for renal failure.

14. What is the most common bacterial organism in bacterial pneumonia?
    a. Streptococcus pneumoniae
    b. Haemophilus influenzae
    c. Klebsiella pneumoniae
    d. Bordetella pertussis

Answer: a. Streptococcus pneumoniae is considered the most common cause of bacterial pneumonia in individuals who are not neonates.

15. What is the major source of pneumonia secondary to a Gram-negative bacterium?
    a. Inhaled spores
    b. Aspiration of vomit
    c. Sinus drainage
    d. Oropharynx

Answer: b. Gram-negative pneumonia comes from the GI tract and the aspiration of GI contents, such as vomit and feces.

16. What symptom/sign would be least likely to be seen in infectious diarrhea?
    a. Diarrhea
    b. Fever
    c. Abdominal pain
    d. Vomiting

Answer: b. Each of these is a typical symptom of infectious diarrhea except for fever, which is less likely to be present in the disorder.

17. What is the most common bacterial cause of gastroenteritis in adults?
    a. Shigella
    b. Salmonella
    c. Campylobacter
    d. Escherichia coli

Answer: c. Campylobacter is the main cause of bacterial gastroenteritis in adults.

18. What is least likely to be a treatment for gastroenteritis?
    a. Oral rehydration solution
    b. Zinc
    c. IV fluids
    d. Antibiotics

Answer: d. Antibiotics are rarely necessary for cases of gastroenteritis, even if the cause is bacterial.

19. What abdominal finding is most specific for peritonitis?
    a. Voluntary guarding
    b. Involuntary guarding
    c. Rebound tenderness
    d. Abdominal rigidity

Answer: d. Abdominal rigidity is a classic finding of peritonitis and will rarely be seen in other causes of abdominal pain.

20. What does the phenomenon of ileus mean?
    a. Spasm of the intestinal tract
    b. Paralysis of the intestinal tract
    c. Perforation of the intestinal tract
    d. Fluid collections in the peritoneal space

Answer: b. Paralysis of the intestinal tract is known as an ileus. There will be an absence of bowel sounds.

21. What finding on culture of the peritoneum suggests that the problem is from a ruptured viscus?
    a. Candida species
    b. Coagulase negative Staphylococcus
    c. Bacillus fragilis
    d. Staphylococcus aureus

Answer: c. A ruptured viscus is likely to grow out Escherichia coli or an anaerobe like Bacillus fragilis because these are bowel organisms. The other choices are skin-related organisms.

22. How long does a person need to have bacterial sinusitis does a person to have "chronic sinusitis"?
    a. 2 weeks

b. 4 weeks

c. 8 weeks

d. 12 weeks

Answer: d. Sinusitis that lasts longer that 12 weeks is considered chronic sinusitis.

23. What is a first-line agent for chronic sinusitis?

a. Amoxicillin

b. Ciprofloxacin

c. Doxycycline

d. Clarithromycin

Answer: a. Amoxicillin is one of the first antibiotics that should be used in cases of acute sinusitis that doesn't respond to watchful waiting.

24. Which of the following types of otitis media is not associated with hearing loss?

a. Acute otitis media

b. Otitis media with effusion

c. Chronic suppurative otitis media

d. None of the above

Answer: d. Each of these can result in hearing loss but of various durations.

25. What is the antibiotic of choice as a first-line agent in acute otitis media?

a. Ciprofloxacin

b. Doxycycline

c. Amoxicillin

d. Cefuroxime

Answer: c. Patients with non-complicated acute otitis media can be treated with amoxicillin.

26. What is the approximate mortality rate in patients who have tuberculosis?

a. 1 percent

b. 5 percent

c. 20 percent

d. 50 percent

Answer: b. Only 10 percent of patients develop active disease and only half of these patients will die from the infection, leading to a 5 percent mortality rate.

27. What is the most common location of extrapulmonary tuberculosis?

a. Lymph nodes

b. Pleura

c. Bone

d. Disseminated

Answer: a. The most common place to have extrapulmonary tuberculosis is the lymph nodes, which will gradually enlarge without pain.

28. How long does it take for an influenza vaccination to take effect?

a. 2 days
b. 7 days
c. 14 days
d. 21 days

Answer: c. It takes two weeks or 14 days to become immune to influenza after receiving the vaccination.

29. In what way are upper respiratory virus infections classified?
    a. By the type of virus that infects the respiratory tract
    b. By the effective treatment of the virus
    c. By the length of time the illness takes to recover (acute versus chronic)
    d. By the area of the body infected by the virus

Answer: d. Upper respiratory infections are classified by the area of the body infected by the virus.

30. What type of upper respiratory tract infection is considered a complication of a URI rather than the URI itself?
    a. Bronchitis
    b. Rhinitis
    c. Laryngitis
    d. Pharyngitis

Answer: a. In general, bronchitis is a complication of a URI and is not actually the URI itself. The others are all types of URIs.

31. About what percentage of babies will develop bronchiolitis from an infection with the respiratory syncytial virus?
    a. 2-3 percent
    b. 8-10 percent
    c. 20-25 percent
    d. 30-35 percent

Answer: a. About 2-3 percent of babies will develop bronchiolitis, often requiring hospitalization and oxygen therapy.

32. What is the incubation period (the time between contracting the virus and getting the symptoms) for respiratory syncytial virus?
    a. 1-2 days
    b. 4-5 days
    c. 6-7 days
    d. 7-10 days

Answer: b. The incubation period for RSV is about 4-5 days (the time between exposure and symptoms).

33. What is not considered a common symptom of viral gastroenteritis?
    a. Headache
    b. Nausea
    c. Vomiting
    d. Watery diarrhea

Answer: a. Typical symptoms seen in viral gastroenteritis include nausea, vomiting, and watery diarrhea. Headaches can be present but these are uncommon.

34. Which type of hepatis is not transmitted by blood and bodily fluids?
    a. Hepatitis B
    b. Hepatitis C
    c. Hepatitis D
    d. Hepatitis E

Answer: d. Hepatitis E is transmitted by means of the fecal-oral route.

35. Which type of hepatitis can be prevented for life with a series of vaccines?
    a. Hepatitis B
    b. Hepatitis C
    c. Hepatitis D
    d. Hepatitis E

Answer: a. Hepatitis B has a 3-shot vaccine that confers a lifelong immunity when given to adults or children.

36. Which hepatitis type has medications that can help clear out the infection when chronic?
    a. Hepatitis A
    b. Hepatitis C
    c. Hepatitis D
    e. Hepatitis E

Answer: b. There is medication that can be given for chronic hepatitis B and chronic hepatitis C that are effective in a certain percentage of cases.

37. Which hepatitis virus is incapable of causing an infection by itself and is just a co-infection with another virus?
    a. Hepatitis A
    b. Hepatitis C
    c. Hepatitis D
    e. Hepatitis E

Answer: c. Hepatitis D is a damaged virus that can only infect a person who has already had an infection with hepatitis B that is active and/or chronic.

38. What is the main way that the Epstein-Barr virus is passed from one person to another?
    a. Saliva
    b. Airborne
    c. Fecal-oral
    d. Blood

Answer: a. The Epstein-Barr virus is only transmitted via saliva.

39. What disease would be considered an underlying disorder in Aspergillosis?
    a. Heart failure

b. COPD

c. Stroke

d. Kidney failure

Answer: b. The patient with COPD has a chronic lung disease that predisposes a patient to having aspergillosis.

40. What is the most common location to find aspergillus infections?
    a. Lungs
    b. Ears
    c. Sinuses
    d. Nailbed

Answer: a. The most common place to find aspergillus is in the lungs. The other places can have an aspergillus infection but are less likely.

41. What is the most common strain of aspergillus causing pulmonary disease?
    a. A. clavatus
    b. A. flavus
    c. A. fumigatus
    d. A. lentulus

Answer: c. The most common strain of aspergillus causing pulmonary disease in humans is Aspergillus fumigatus.

42. Which type of histoplasmosis is considered the rarest type?
    a. Acute pulmonary histoplasmosis
    b. Chronic pulmonary histoplasmosis
    c. Ocular histoplasmosis syndrome
    d. Progressive disseminated histoplasmosis

Answer: c. The rarest form of histoplasmosis is called ocular histoplasmosis syndrome, which involves an infection of the eyes.

43. Where is Histoplasma not usually found in the environment?
    a. Soil
    b. Bird droppings
    c. Bat guano
    d. Lake or stream water

Answer: d. The main places for Histoplasma is soil, bird droppings, and bat guano.

44. What happens to the lymph nodes after histoplasmosis heals?
    a. They remain enlarged
    b. They become calcified
    c. They regress to become small nodules
    d. They proliferate to form multiple lymph nodes that are normal in size

Answer: b. After a histoplasmosis infection, the lymph nodes become calcified and can erode into the airways, leading to hemoptysis.

45. What is not considered a predisposing factor for getting cryptococcosis?
    a. Diabetes mellitus
    b. Corticosteroid use
    c. HIV disease
    d. Lymphoma

Answer: a. Each of these is a risk factor for cryptococcosis except for diabetes mellitus.

46. What is not a clinical syndrome seen in cryptococcal disease in humans?
    a. Cutaneous cryptococcosis
    b. Cryptococcal meningitis
    c. Cryptococcal hepatitis
    d. Pulmonary cryptococcosis

Answer: c. Each of these is a type of clinical cryptococcosis except for cryptococcal hepatitis.

47. Which organism is least likely to cause cryptococcal disease in humans?
    a. Cryptococcus neoformans
    b. Cryptococcus albidus
    c. Cryptococcus gattii
    d. Cryptococcus grubii

Answer: b. The least common type of human cryptococcosis is Cryptococcus albidus. The other choices are more likely to cause cryptococcal disease.

48. What is the most sensitive way to identify Cryptococcal meningitis?
    a. Antigen testing of the CSF
    b. CSF culture
    c. India staining of CSF fluid
    d. Antibody testing of CSF testing

Answer: a. Antigen testing of CSF can be used as a sensitive method of detecting cryptococcal meningitis.

49. Where do the malarial organisms reproduce after infecting the human host?
    a. Liver
    b. Bloodstream
    c. GI tract
    d. Brain

Answer: a. The organisms causing malaria travel to the liver where they reproduce and get sent out to the bloodstream.

50. What is the most common symptom complex seen in toxoplasmosis infections?
    a. Myalgias
    b. No symptoms

c. Lymphadenitis

d. Seizures

Answer: b. Toxoplasmosis rarely causes any symptoms in the immunocompetent person.

51. What is not considered a way to contract toxoplasmosis?
    a. Exposure to cat feces
    b. Eating poorly cooked food
    c. Airborne droplets when coughing
    d. In utero exposure

Answer: c. Toxoplasmosis can be contracted through each of these exposures except for airborne droplets from coughing as it is not passed from person to person in that way.

52. What is the most effective test for leishmaniasis?
    a. PCR test of blood
    b. Direct tissue staining
    c. Direct agglutination test
    d. ELISA test

Answer: a. The PCR test is easy, sensitive, and specific. The direct tissue testing is sensitive but painful, and both the direct agglutination test and the ELISA test are not very accurate.

53. Which protozoal disease is not transmitted by an insect bite or sting?
    a. Leishmaniasis
    b. Malaria
    c. Toxoplasmosis
    d. African sleeping sickness

Answer: c. Of the listed choices, all are caused by the bite or sting of an insect except for toxoplasmosis, which is not related to an insect vector.

54. Which is not a symptom of the second stage of African trypanosomiasis?
    a. Insomnia
    b. Confusion
    c. Poor coordination
    d. Arthralgias

Answer: d. Arthralgias are seen in the first stage of the disease, while CNS findings can be seen in the second stage of the disease.

55. Which protozoal infection stems from the bite of the kissing bug?
    a. Chagas disease
    b. African sleeping sickness
    c. Leishmaniasis
    d. Giardiasis

Answer: a. Chagas disease is caused by the bite of an infected kissing bug. It is also called American trypanosomiasis.

56. What protozoal disease is also called African trypanosomiasis?
    a. Chagas disease
    b. Malaria
    c. African sleeping sickness
    d. Leishmaniasis

Answer: c. The disease called African trypanosomiasis is also called African sleeping sickness.

57. Which is considered the most accurate test for Chagas disease?
    a. Polymerase chain reaction
    b. Direct visualization of blood smear
    c. ELISA testing
    d. Radio-immunoassay testing

Answer: b. The best way to evaluate a patient for Chagas disease is to either do a direct visualization or a xenodiagnosis. The other tests are not as accurate for the disease.

58. What is the duration of the disease in untreated Giardia lamblia infections?
    a. 2 weeks
    b. 4 weeks
    c. 6 weeks
    d. Indefinite

Answer: c. The total duration of untreated disease in giardiasis is about six weeks and will often resolve on its own.

59. What feature is common to most tapeworm species?
    a. Lifespan entirely within one host individual.
    b. Neurological disease because of brain involvement
    c. The presence of four suckers on the head of the worm
    d. The ingestion of raw pork causing the disease

Answer: c. A feature common to all tapeworm species except for fish tapeworm is the presence of four suckers on the head of the worm allowing it to attach to the GI wall.

60. What is the most common initial symptom seen in patients suffering from ascariasis?
    a. Diarrhea
    b. Dyspnea
    c. Abdominal distention
    d. Abdominal pain

Answer: b. Dyspnea and fever are the initial symptoms present with ascariasis. The other symptoms are secondary ones.

61. What is involved with Loeffler's syndrome in ascariasis?
    a. Pulmonary infiltrates and eosinophilia
    b. Intestinal obstruction
    c. Diarrhea and hematochezia
    d. Hepatomegaly

Answer: a. Loeffler's syndrome involves pulmonary infiltrates and eosinophilia in ascariasis cases.

62. What type of filariasis leads to river blindness?
    a. Oncherocera volvulus
    b. Wuchereria bancrofti
    c. Mansonella streptocerca
    d. Loa loa

Answer: a. An infestation of Oncherocera volvulus infests the subcutaneous tissues and leads to river blindness.

63. In which body area does serous cavity filariasis mainly take residence?
    a. Pleural space
    b. Pericardial space
    c. Peritoneal space
    d. Retroperitoneal space

Answer: c. The serous cavity that involves this type of filariasis is the peritoneal space, leading to abdominal pain and distention.

64. What is the best way to detect most cases of filariasis?
    a. Antibody testing of serum
    b. Direct visualization of the worms or eggs in the stool
    c. Antigen testing of the stool
    d. Direct visualization of the larvae in the bloodstream

Answer: d. Direct visualization of the larvae in the bloodstream can detect many cases of filariasis except those that don't travel through the bloodstream.

65. What is the main symptom seen in infestations with scabies?
    a. Intense itching
    b. Red macules
    c. Lymphadenopathy
    d. Diffuse burrows

Answer: a. The main symptom seen in scabies infestations is intense itching. Patients will have a papular skin rash and rarely will have occasional burrows under the skin from the mite's travels.

66. Which of the following is an oral medication for scabies versus a topical medication?
    a. Permethrin
    b. Crotamiton
    c. Lindane
    d. Ivermectin

Answer: d. Of the choices of medications for scabies, only Ivermectin is an oral medication. The others are topical anti-scabies agents.

67. What common disease is also referred to as "crabs"?
    a. Scabies

b. Pediculosis pubis

c. Pediculosis capitis

d. Pediculosis corporis

Answer: b. Pediculosis pubis is a type of parasitic infestation that is commonly referred to as "crabs".

68. What causes itching in cases of pediculosis pubis?
    a. Hypersensitivity to saliva of the insect
    b. Burrowing of the insect in the skin
    c. Hypersensitivity of the insect's feces
    d. Irritation of the insects crawling on the skin

Answer: a. The intense itching seen in the disease stems from a hypersensitivity reaction to the insect's saliva.

69. What is the best way to make an accurate diagnosis of pediculosis capitis?
    a. Visualization of nits
    b. Antigen testing of blood
    c. Antibody testing of blood
    d. Visualization of adult lice

Answer: d. It takes visualization of adult lice to make the diagnosis. There are no blood tests for the disorder and nits alone do not confirm the diagnosis.

70. How long do adult head lice live when not in contact with the body?
    a. One day
    b. Three days
    c. Five days
    d. Ten days

Answer: b. The live louse can live outside the body for a total of about three days before they die.

71. Which is a popular topical antibiotic for skin or nasal infections caused by Staphylococcus aureus and that has minimal allergic potential?
    a. Mupirocin
    b. Penicillin
    c. Trimethoprim/sulfamethoxazole
    d. Tetracycline

Answer: a. Mupirocin has good activity against Staphylococcus aureus but is not absorbed so it has minimal allergic potential.

72. Which antibiotic carries a high risk of photosensitivity, involving a rash or sunburn when exposed to the sun while taking the drug?
    a. Erythromycin
    b. Tetracycline
    c. Penicillin
    d. Bactrim

Answer: b. Tetracycline and drugs of this class will carry a risk of a photosensitivity reaction when taken and being exposed to the sun in some patients.

73. Why is diarrhea a common complication of taking broad-spectrum antibiotics?
    a. It causes malabsorption of fat in the small intestine
    b. The antibiotic causes stomach and small intestinal toxicity
    c. The antibiotic destroys normal gastrointestinal flora, contributing to pathogenic overgrowth
    d. The antibiotic makes the patient more sensitive to viral gastroenteritis

Answer: c. The antibiotic can cause diarrhea by destroying normal GI flora, contributing to the overgrowth of pathogenic bacteria that can cause diarrhea.

74. Which generation of cephalosporin has good anti-Pseudomonas activity?
    a. First-generation
    b. Second-generation
    c. Third-generation
    d. Fourth-generation

Answer: d. Fourth-generation cephalosporins have specific activity against Pseudomonas.

75. To which classification of drugs does silver sulfadiazine belong?
    a. Sulfonamides
    b. Quinolones
    c. Tetracyclines
    d. Macrolides

Answer: a. Silver sulfadiazine belongs to the sulfonamide classification of drugs.

76. What is a major difference between antiviral drugs and antibacterial agents?
    a. Antiviral drugs are all able to kill the virus, while antibacterial drugs may not kill the bacterium.
    b. Antiviral drugs cannot kill the virus, while antibacterial drugs can kill the bacterium.
    c. Antiviral drugs have more toxicity than antibacterial drugs.
    d. There are more side effects with antiviral drugs than antibacterial drugs.

Answer: b. Antiviral drugs cannot kill the virus, while antibacterial drugs can kill the bacterium in some cases (depending on the classification of antibacterial drug).

77. Which influenza drug is no longer recommended for the treatment of influenza because of significant resistances?
    a. Zanamivir
    b. Amantadine
    c. Oseltamivir
    d. Acyclovir

Answer: b. Amantadine was once a commonly-used drug for the treatment of influenza but, because of resistances, it is no longer recommended for the prevention or treatment of influenza.

78. Zanamivir (Relenza) is a drug used for the treatment of influenza. How much shorter is the duration of symptoms of the flu if the patient takes the drug versus not taking the drug?
    a. One day
    b. Three days
    c. Five days
    d. Seven days

Answer: a. The duration of the disease is only reduced by one day if the patient takes the drug so it isn't recommended in the healthy patient.

79. Many drugs for influenza are neuraminidase inhibitors. What does this do to the viral particles to prevent or treat infections?
    a. It prevents viral attachment to the cell
    b. It blocks the removal of the viral coat in the cell
    c. It blocks the replication of the virus's RNA or DNA
    d. It blocks the release of the newly-made virus particles from infected cells

Answer: d. The drugs that act as neuraminidase inhibitors are effective in preventing the release of newly-made virus particles from previously infected cells.

80. What is the main antiviral drug used to treat herpes zoster?
    a. Adefovir
    b. Famciclovir
    c. Interferon
    d. Peramivir

Answer: b. Famciclovir is the main antiviral drug used to treat herpes zoster infections.

81. What major toxicity is seen in patients taking oral terbinafine?
    a. Renal toxicity
    b. Hepatotoxicity
    c. Neurotoxicity
    d. Bone marrow toxicity

Answer: b. Terbinafine or Lamisil, if taken orally, can cause hepatotoxicity, requiring the need to check liver function tests periodically while on the drug.

82. Which common antifungal drug can be used orally or intravenously for a variety of fungal infections?
    a. Terbinafine
    b. Miconazole
    c. Fluconazole
    d. Clotrimazole

Answer: c. Fluconazole can be used intravenously or orally for many different fungal infections.

83. Why is ketoconazole not a first-line drug for systemic fungal infections?
    a. It carries a greater risk of hepatotoxicity compared to related drugs.
    b. It has an unpredictable pharmacokinetic pattern.

c. It cannot be used orally and must be intravenous.

d. It doesn't work on the immunosuppressed patient.

Answer: a. Ketoconazole is not used systemically as often because it will cause a greater chance of developing hepatotoxicity compared to other drugs of its class.

84. Which malarial drug has the highest rate of resistances?
    a. Chloroquine
    b. Quinidine
    c. Amodiaquine
    d. Pyrimethamine

Answer: a. Chloroquine has the highest rate of resistances.

85. What anti-malarial drug is only used in the prevention of malaria but cannot be used in an acute infection?
    a. Sulfadoxine
    b. Sulfamethoxypyridazine
    c. Pyrimethamine
    d. Proguanil

Answer: d. Only proguanil is recommended solely for the prevention of malaria as it cannot treat active infections.

86. What antimalarial drug probably shouldn't be given to psychiatric patients because of a high degree of psychiatric side effects?
    a. Sulfadoxine
    b. Mefloquine
    c. Pyrimethamine
    d. Proguanil

Answer: b. Mefloquine has many psychiatric side effects so it should be given with caution in patients who already have psychiatric disease.

87. What anti-parasitic drug can be used in both African sleeping sickness and river blindness?
    a. Eflornithine
    b. Nifurtimox
    c. Suramin
    d. Melarsoprol

Answer: c. Suramin is used as a second-line agent for first-stage African sleeping sickness and for the treatment of river blindness.

88. What is the name given to antihelminthic drugs used to kill worms of all types?
    a. Vermifuges
    b. Vermicides
    c. Anthelmintics
    d. Ascaricides

Answer: b. Vermicides are antihelminthic drugs that kill worms of all types as opposed to stunning the worms or killing only certain types of worms as is the case with ascaricides.

89. Which antihelminthic drug is the most effective in killing most kinds of helminths?
    a. Albendazole
    b. Mebendazole
    c. Suramin
    d. Niclosamide

Answer: a. Albendazole is effective in killing a variety of helminths, which isn't the case for the other antihelminthic drugs listed.

90. What is considered the first-line treatment for head lice?
    a. Malathion
    b. Piperonyl butoxide
    c. Lindane
    d. Pyrethrins

Answer: d. Pyrethrins are considered the first-line treatment for head lice, particularly in children.

91. What anti-lice treatment is an oral drug versus a topical drug?
    a. Malathion
    b. Ivermectin
    c. Lindane
    d. Pyrethrin

Answer: b. Ivermectin is a second-line treatment for lice that is the only oral medication used to treat head lice.

92. The 65-year-old male patient has a positive blood culture associated with discrete left lower quadrant tenderness. What is the most likely source of the infection?
    a. Appendicitis
    b. Pyelonephritis
    c. Diverticulitis
    d. Prostatic abscess

Answer: c. The finding of LLQ abdominal tenderness is most suggestive of sepsis secondary to diverticulitis and a ruptured diverticulum.

93. If a patient has suspected sepsis from a possible infected central line site, what percentage of the time will there be evidence of a local infection at the site?
    a. 10 percent
    b. 50 percent
    c. 75 percent
    d. 95 percent

Answer: b. Only 50 percent of the time would there be an actual noticeable infection at the site of a central line infection leading to sepsis.

94. What type of blood vessel line is most likely to lead to septicemia and sepsis?
    a. Intraosseous
    b. Arterial
    c. Peripheral venous
    d. Central venous

Answer: d. The most common site that will lead to sepsis is a central venous line. The others are least likely to result in a bloodborne infection.

95. What would an ultrasound of the abdomen be most helpful in diagnosing when evaluating the septic patient for an abdominal cause of sepsis?
    a. Abdominal abscess
    b. Appendicitis
    c. Diverticulitis
    d. Biliary obstruction

Answer: d. The ultrasound of the abdomen is usually only successful in diagnosing biliary obstruction and is less effective in diagnosing any other intraabdominal source of septicemia.

96. What is not considered an end-result of the cytokine release seen in sepsis?
    a. Tachypnea
    b. Liver failure
    c. Adrenal failure
    d. Acute renal dysfunction

Answer: c. The main things seen as a part of the cytokine release seen in sepsis is tachypnea (followed by pulmonary dysfunction), liver failure, and renal dysfunction. Adrenal failure is not a part of the problem seen in sepsis.

97. How long should the average patient with sepsis be treated with antibiotic therapy?
    a. 5 days
    b. 9 days
    c. 14 days
    d. 21 days

Answer: c. The patient with sepsis needs to be treated for approximately 14 days with antibiotics after the cause has been identified and surgical intervention has taken place.

98. What antibiotic is not considered to be a possible choice in the management of intraabdominal infections causing sepsis?
    a. Cefotaxime
    b. Metronidazole
    c. Aminoglycosides
    d. Clindamycin

Answer: a. Choices of antibiotics for intraabdominal or pelvic infections causing sepsis include imipenem, piperacillin-tazobactam, meropenem, tigecycline, or ampicillin-sulbactam (as monotherapy) or dual therapy with either metronidazole or clindamycin plus an aminoglycoside, levofloxacin, or aztreonam.

99. Which organism is not to be specifically considered in cases of instrument-related urosepsis?
    a. Pseudomonas aeruginosa
    b. Klebsiella pneumoniae
    c. Serratia
    d. Enterobacter

Answer: b. Each of these should be considered in instrument-related urosepsis except for Klebsiella pneumoniae, which is not a likely cause of this problem.

100. What vancomycin-resistant organism is emerging as being the result of overuse of the drug?
    a. Staphylococcus
    b. Enterobacter
    c. Enterococcus
    d. Klebsiella

Answer: c. VRE or vancomycin-resistant Enterococcus faecium is the organism emerging from overuse of vancomycin.

101. Which cause of sepsis would require a course of antibiotic therapy lasting longer than three weeks?
    a. Pyelonephritis
    b. Prostatitis
    c. Diverticulitis
    d. Liver abscess

Answer: d. Liver abscesses are difficult to treatment for longer than three weeks in order to affect a cure.

102. Which types of cells are least likely to be actively infected by the HIV virus?
    a. Macrophages
    b. Dendritic cells
    c. Helper T cells
    d. Histiocytes

Answer: d. Each of these cells is infected by the HIV virus except for histiocytes, which are not generally seen as infected immune cells in HIV disease.

103. What is the ribonucleic acid structure of the HIV virus?
    a. Single-stranded RNA
    b. Double-stranded RNA
    c. Single-stranded DNA
    d. Double-stranded DNA

Answer: a. The HIV virus is a single-stranded RNA virus that is a positive-sense ribonucleic acid.

104. What is the first virally-encoded enzyme utilized after the HIV virus enters a cell it has infected?

a. DNA polymerase

b. Ribonuclease

c. Reverse transcriptase

d. Integrase

Answer: c. Reverse transcriptase turns the viral RNA (single-stranded) into a double-stranded DNA particle and is the first enzyme used by the virus after infection.

105. Which subtype of HIV is the most prevalent in terms of numbers of infected people?
    a. Subtype A
    b. Subtype B
    c. Subtype C
    d. Subtype D

Answer: c. Subtype C accounts for 47 percent of HIV infections. It is mainly found in Africa and Asia. The other subtypes are much less common.

106. Which HIV test is not considered a confirmatory test for the disease and is, in fact, a screening test?
    a. ELISA
    b. Western-blot
    c. IFA
    d. PCR

Answer: a. The ELISA test (enzyme-linked immunosorbent assay) is a screening test for HIV and is not a confirmatory test.

107. The HIV-exposed patient is tested immediately after being exposed and three more times after that. When is not a typical time for retesting of the blood after an exposure?
    a. Six weeks
    b. Three months
    c. Six months
    d. One year

Answer: d. The blood is tested at regular intervals up until six months. If the test is negative at six months, the patient is not likely to be infected and does not require subsequent follow-up.

108. What is the most common virus-related cancer linked to patients who have AIDS?
    a. Primary central nervous system lymphoma
    b. Kaposi's sarcoma
    c. Cervical cancer
    d. Burkitt's lymphoma

Answer: b. Kaposi's sarcoma is the most common viral-related cancer linked to patients who have AIDS, occurring in up to 20 percent of patients.

109. What virus is linked to Kaposi's sarcoma and lymphoma in AIDS patients?
    a. Herpes simplex I
    b. Human papillomavirus

c. Hepatitis A

d. Herpesvirus 8

Answer: d. Infections with herpesvirus 8 can cause lymphoma and Kaposi's sarcoma in AIDS patients.

110. What is the route of transmission for HIV disease that leads to the highest chance of getting an infection?
    a. Receptive anal intercourse
    b. Blood transfusion
    c. Sharing dirty needles
    d. Needlestick in the workplace

Answer: b. Blood transfusions have a 90 percent chance of developing an infection with HIV if the blood is infected with the virus.

111. What is the most common way to get the HIV infection?
    a. Sexual intercourse
    b. IV drug use
    c. Blood transfusion
    d. Needlestick

Answer: a. HIV is transmitted to a greater degree through blood transfusions, however, blood is screened before it is given. Thus, the most common way of getting the virus is through sexual intercourse with an infected person.

112. What type of cancer is linked to having an infection with gonorrhea?
    a. Uterine
    b. Ovarian
    c. Testicular
    d. Prostate

Answer: d. Having gonorrhea in life predisposes men to developing prostate cancer for reasons that are not clear.

113. The treatment of choice for gonorrhea is ceftriaxone and what other antibiotic?
    a. Erythromycin
    b. Azithromycin
    c. Tetracycline
    d. Ciprofloxacin

Answer: b. Ceftriaxone is combined with azithromycin to cover for gonorrhea and chlamydia, which often coexist in the same person.

114. The lack of treatment of what sexually transmitted disease can lead to trachoma and blindness?
    a. Chlamydia
    b. Gonorrhea
    c. Syphilis
    d. Human papillomavirus

Answer: a. Untreated chlamydia can lead to a roughening of the inner surface of the eyelids (trachoma) and blindness, particularly in developing countries.

115. What is the current screening recommendation(s) for syphilis?
    a. Screening all women under the age of 25 years annually.
    b. Screening sexually active men and women every 3-5 years.
    c. Screening homosexual and bisexual men under the age of 30 years.
    d. Screening all newly pregnant women.

Answer: d. Screening is currently recommended for all women at the time of their first prenatal visit.

116. Which stage of syphilis is represented as a chancre on the penis or cervix?
    a. Primary
    b. Secondary
    c. Latent
    d. Tertiary

Answer: a. A chancre is present primarily in primary syphilis and not in any other stage of syphilis.

117. Which stage of syphilis is the patient not infectious?
    a. Primary
    b. Secondary
    c. Latent
    d. Tertiary

Answer: d. The patient with tertiary syphilis will be symptomatic but will not be infectious.

118. What treatment can be given in neurosyphilis to reverse the neurological damage?
    a. IV penicillin given for three weeks
    b. Doxycycline orally for three weeks
    c. IM ceftriaxone for four weeks
    d. No antibiotic can reverse the damage caused by neurosyphilis

Answer: d. Any of the above choices can be used for neurosyphilis but no treatment will treat the preexisting damage to the brain.

119. Which type of cancer is almost exclusively secondary to a human papillomavirus infection?
    a. Vagina
    b. Cervix
    c. Anal
    d. Penile

Answer: b. Most cases of cervical cancer stem from an HPV infection, with two strains primarily accounting for the cancer.

120. Which type of cancer is not highly linked to an infection with human papillomavirus?
    a. Anal
    b. Penile
    c. Laryngeal

d. Ovarian

Answer: d. Each of these cancers is highly linked to an HPV infection except for ovarian cancer.

121. Which is the most common STI in the US?
    a. Herpes simplex-2
    b. Genital warts
    c. Gonorrhea
    d. Chlamydia

Answer: a. Herpes simplex-2 is the most common STI in the US; however, HPV is the most common STI in the world.

122. What country has the highest rate of dengue fever cases?
    a. India
    b. Cambodia
    c. Indonesia
    d. Philippines

Answer: c. The greatest risk of dengue fever and death from complications occurs in Indonesia.

123. What percentage of patients with dengue fever will have symptoms?
    a. 20 percent
    b. 50 percent
    c. 75 percent
    d. 95 percent

Answer: a. Only about 20 percent of patients who contract the virus will have symptoms of the disorder. The others will be asymptomatic or may have only mild symptoms.

124. What lab diagnosis is not necessarily seen in severe hemorrhagic fever?
    a. Increased liver function tests
    b. Thrombocytosis
    c. Hypoalbuminemia
    d. Leukopenia

Answer: b. Patients with dengue will have thrombocytopenia instead of thrombocytosis.

125. What characteristic of the lesions of leprosy indicate that the skin lesions are from this disease versus other rashes?
    a. The presence of red papules
    b. The lesions are mainly on the fingers and toes
    c. The lesions are anesthetized and numb
    d. The lesions will weep clear fluid

Answer: c. A characteristic of the lesions of leprosy are that they are anesthetized and numb due to nerve damage of the affected area.

126. The patient is found to have multibacillary leprosy and is treated with combination therapy using three drugs. How long must they be treated in order to affect a cure?

a. Two weeks
b. Three months
c. Six months
d. One year

Answer: d. The patient with multibacillary disease is treated for one year with three medications in order to affect a cure.

127. What is the percent mortality rate of untreated rabies that reaches the CNS?
    a. 10 percent
    b. 35 percent
    c. 70 percent
    d. 100 percent

Answer: d. Patients who contract rabies that reaches the CNS have a 100 percent mortality rate once the disease reaches the CNS.

128. How many doses of the rabies vaccine need to be given as part of post-exposure therapy for the disease?
    a. One
    b. Two
    c. Three
    d. Four

Answer: d. A total of four doses of the vaccine given on day 1, 3, 7, and 14 should be given to patients with a high chance of being exposed to the virus.

129. Which rare disease is not cause by a bacterial organism?
    a. Typhus
    b. Rabies
    c. Leprosy
    d. Trachoma

Answer: b. Each of these is caused by a bacterial organism except for rabies, which is a viral disease.

130. What is the recommendation around treating a patient with trachoma?
    a. The patient cannot be treated as the disease is immune to antibiotics.
    b. The patient should be treated with antibiotics as well as their sexual contacts.
    c. The patient and all significant contacts should be given antibiotics.
    d. Only the patient should receive antibiotics.

Answer: c. The patient and all significant contacts need antibiotics as the disease can be spread through casual contact, flies, contaminated water, and clothing. Mass community treatment is recommended when the prevalence of the disease reaches 10 percent or more.

131. What is the treatment of choice for people who have trachoma?
    a. Single dose of azithromycin
    b. Two weeks of topical tetracycline
    c. Two weeks of topical erythromycin

d. Single dose of doxycycline

Answer: a. The treatment of choice for trachoma is a single dose of azithromycin.

132. What vector is not common for typhus fever?
    a. Fleas
    b. Mosquitos
    c. Chiggers
    d. Body lice

Answer: b. Any type of the above vectors can lead to typhus except for mosquitos, which are not vectors for the disease.

133. Which antibiotic is most effective in treating MRSA?
    a. Clindamycin
    b. Vancomycin
    c. Tetracycline
    d. Linezolid

Answer: d. Linezolid will eradicate MRSA in about 87 percent of patients with very little resistances found in the community.

134. What type of infection is pneumocystis pneumonia (PCP)?
    a. Viral
    b. Bacterial
    c. Fungal
    d. Parasitic

Answer: c. A yeast-like fungus is the main cause of pneumocystis pneumonia in immunocompromised hosts.

135. Where is the pneumocystis organism normally found in the healthy human host?
    a. Upper respiratory tract
    b. Lower respiratory tract
    c. GI tract
    d. Not commonly found in a healthy human

Answer: d. There is no place on the body or in the body of immunocompetent hosts that pneumocystis can be discovered.

136. What is not considered a complication of a Clostridium difficile infection?
    a. Toxic megacolon
    b. Pseudomembranous colitis
    c. Colonic abscesses
    d. Septicemia

Answer: c. Each of these can be complications of Clostridium difficile colitis except for colonic abscesses, which tend not to form in the disease.

137. What is not a typical way to diagnose a Clostridium difficile infection of the bowels?

a. Stool culture
b. Antibody testing of blood
c. PCR test of the stool
d. Toxin test of the stool

Answer: b. Tests primarily on the stool are the preferred mechanism of identifying a clostridium infection. Antibody testing will not be helpful in diagnosing this disorder.

138. What antibiotic is not used in the treatment of Clostridium difficile infection?
    a. Clindamycin
    b. Metronidazole
    c. Vancomycin
    d. Fidaxomicin

Answer: a. Clindamycin is not an effective treatment for Clostridium difficile infections.

139. In a patient suspected of having active CMV disease, which is the least likely way of evaluating whether the patient has an active infection?
    a. DNA testing of blood
    b. Antigen testing of blood
    c. Urine culture for the virus
    d. Tissue biopsy of suspected infection

Answer: c. Any of these will be effective in detecting active disease except for a urine culture, which will not detect active disease but will represent viral shedding instead.

140. Which CMV infection is almost exclusively seen in AIDS patients?
    a. Hepatitis
    b. Meningitis
    c. Pharyngitis
    d. Retinitis

Answer: d. CMV retinitis is primarily seen in AIDS patients who are immunosuppressed.

Made in the USA
Las Vegas, NV
25 June 2024

91488831R00090